NURSES WORK: AN ANALYSIS OF THE UK LABOUR MARKET

Nurses Work: An Analysis of the UK Nursing Labour Market

JAMES BUCHAN
Reader, Department of Management & Social Science,
Queen Margaret College, Edinburgh

IAN SECCOMBE
Associate Fellow of the Institute for Employment Studies,
Brighton

GABRIELLE SMITH
Research Fellow of the Institute for Employment Studies
Brighton

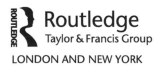
Routledge
Taylor & Francis Group
LONDON AND NEW YORK

First published 1998 by Ashgate Publishing

Reissued 2018 by Routledge
2 Park Square, Milton Park, Abingdon, Oxon, OX14 4RN
711 Third Avenue, New York, NY 10017, USA

Routledge is an imprint of the Taylor & Francis Group, an informa business

Publisher's Note
The publisher has gone to great lengths to ensure the quality of this reprint but points out that some imperfections in the original copies may be apparent.

Disclaimer
The publisher has made every effort to trace copyright holders and welcomes correspondence from those they have been unable to contact.

A Library of Congress record exists under LC control number: 98771462

ISBN 13: 978-1-138-32658-3 (hbk)
ISBN 13: 978-1-138-32659-0 (pbk)
ISBN 13: 978-0-429-44979-6 (ebk)

Contents

List of Figures

List of Tables

Acknowledgements

This book would not have been possible without access to the data and information provided by the nurses who have contributed to the annual surveys supported by the Royal College of Nursing. Our thanks are to the tens of thousands of nurses who have taken time out of their busy schedules to participate over the years, sustaining a consistently high response rate. The support of the Royal College of Nursing, and the commitment of its General Secretary, Christine Hancock, and its Director of Labour Relations, Phil Gray, have also been vital to the continued development of the surveys as a unique source of information on the nursing workforce in the United Kingdom. We acknowledge the other staff at IES who have contributed as authors to one or more of the annual surveys over the years. Richard Waite, Rosemary Hutt, Jane Thomas, John Stock, Jane Ball, Adrian Patch, Charles Jackson and Monica Haynes have all made a contribution. Finally, we would like to thank Carol Barber for helping to shape the final product.

James Buchan
Ian Seccombe
Gabrielle Smith

December 1997

Foreword

Published in the midst of one of the worst shortage of nurses in the history of the National Health Service, this book is a timely reminder that we rarely learn from history. As we celebrate 50 years of NHS nursing and the huge contribution that nurses have made to the National Health Service, we also mark a 50 year history characterised by a lack of investment in planning the nursing workforce.

Nurses are by far the largest workforce in the health service. Yet poor workforce planning is perhaps inevitable when nursing is still thought of by some as an instinctive, caring job fit for any 'good woman'. Nursing has long suffered from myth making, but none worse that the myth which claims nurses are not interested in developing their skills as expert members of the health care team.

Employers, governments, research findings - and most importantly, patients - recognise the value of expert nurses. They realise that nurses provide cost effective, high quality care. But while everyone appreciates the value of expert nurses, we are still failing to invest properly in the planning, education and training of the nursing workforce. If we value the contribution that nurses make to the NHS, then we need to value their careers. It is impossible to do one without the other.

This book sounds a warning bell for the NHS. It paints a very clear picture of the challenges ahead, plugging many of the information gaps which previously made it impossible to pull together a comprehensive overview of the nursing labour market. Yet unlike other warning bells, this time we need to learn from history. The stakes are too high if we ignore it.

Christine Hancock, General Secretary of the Royal College of Nursing

1 Introduction

Recent years have seen significant changes in the labour market behaviour of registered nurses[1] and in their patterns of employment and career opportunities. The growth of employment outside the National Health Service (NHS), the emphasis on developing community based care, and organisational change in the NHS acute sector, have all impacted on the nursing labour market, as have broader economic and societal factors.

The nursing workforce is the core of the health services, both in the NHS and the private sector. With over half a million registered nurses in work, nursing is currently the largest source of professional employment for females in the United Kingdom (UK)[2]. The NHS nursing paybill, estimated by the Review Body to be £7,857 million in 1996-97, accounts for 3 per cent of all public sector expenditure. For such a large and important group, nursing has received comparatively scant attention in terms of evaluating employment policy and practice.

Over the decades there have been a series of often sterile, and sometimes ill informed, debates about trends in nursing employment, the 'right' number of nurses to recruit, and issues of nurses' pay, morale and labour market behaviour. The aims of this book are to provide a definitive profile of the UK nursing workforce, to highlight some of the issues facing nurses at work, and to present a critique of approaches to nurse workforce planning in UK nursing. In order to achieve this, the book:

- establishes the current profile of the UK nursing labour market;

- identifies key trends in labour market behaviour and career paths of nurses;

- highlights changes in non-NHS employment;

- identifies gaps in official data provision;

- assesses implications for policy makers of likely key trends and other labour market related issues (*eg* end of 'job for life', changes in demand, flexible working, ageing workforce, growth of new labour markets, organisational change *etc.*); and

1

- undertakes supply modelling to test different assumptions on intakes to pre-registration nurse education and future trends in staffing.

The book makes use of data from official sources, but also draws heavily from the various studies undertaken by the Institute for Employment Studies (IES), and commissioned by the Royal College of Nursing (RCN). The Institute has conducted twelve national surveys of registered nurses for the RCN since the mid 1980s. These surveys provide a unique source of data on the experiences and opinions of nurses in the UK. They have been conducted during years of significant change in nurses' labour market behaviour and in their patterns of employment and career opportunities.

Some of the key changes which provide the backdrop for the book are the NHS reforms, changes to NHS nurses' pay determination and employee relations, and the restructuring of nurse education in the UK ('Project 2000'). The effects of these changes will be considered in detail in subsequent chapters. Their main features are discussed below.

1.1 The National Health Service reforms

The 1988 review of the NHS, which led to the passing of the NHS and Community Care Act 1990 and to the implementation of the health reforms in 1991, was a political reaction to a series of high profile NHS resourcing problems. A number of these problems related to nurse staffing, such as the shortage of specialist nurses at a hospital in Birmingham. Solving the problems of skills shortages and securing improvements in employee 'productivity' became central tenets of the NHS reforms.

The NHS is a labour intensive industry: it is estimated that salaries and wages of staff directly employed by the NHS represented two-thirds (64 per cent) of health authorities' gross revenue expenditure in 1994 (Office of Health Economics, 1995). The workforce is large (more than one million are employed in several hundred establishments), and is heavily unionised with several powerful professional and generalist unions. Nursing represents the largest element of the NHS workforce, with more than 350,000 registered nurses in its employment.

Nursing is also labour intensive, and the pre-reform service relied on centralised national negotiations of terms and conditions of employment, with local activity primarily being 'hiring and firing' and dealing with individual grievances. Other activities (for example, training and development, workforce planning) varied markedly in depth and effect at local level (see Buchan and Seccombe, 1994).

The NHS reforms of the 1990s had been preceded by the 'Griffiths' reforms of NHS management. The Griffiths' reforms in 1983 had replaced consensus management with general management. A team of four senior officers (nurse, administrator, doctor and accountant) responsible for managing jointly each District Health Authority (DHA) were replaced with a single general manager who had overall accountability and responsibility at DHA level for the management of services. The implementation of the Griffiths' recommendations also marked the beginning of an increased role for the personnel function in the DHA.

The process of change in the NHS, begun by Griffiths, was accelerated by the publication of the White Paper *Working for Patients* in 1989. The White Paper contained three central elements:

- decentralisation of managerial responsibility (including a move from central to local pay determination);

- the introduction of the internal market ('purchaser/provider' split); and

- the establishment of self-governing NHS trusts replacing the DHA as the 'employer'.

These three elements had significant implications for the management of labour costs and of the NHS workforce. One of the driving forces behind the reforms was to improve cost containment. Staffing, as the major element of expenditure, constituted an obvious area for improvement in terms of 'value for money'. However, there was little specific guidance in the content of the White Paper, or the subsequent NHS and Community Care Act 1990, as to how these changes were to be implemented. There was little mention of nursing or other non-medical employment issues, and few considerations of employment practice. Beyond the general assumptions built into the reforms that devolution, decentralisation and flexibility should be articles of faith in the post-reform management of NHS staff, there was no detailed formula for change. Indeed, such an approach would have cut across the grain of the reforms, which places the emphasis on local management's 'right' and responsibility to manage.

The election of a new Labour government in 1997 marked an end to almost 20 years of Conservative control. At the time of writing it is clear that Labour will initiate significant changes in health policy, but that organisational 'flexibility' and decentralised decision making are likely to remain as key features of the NHS, as will continued pressure to contain costs.

1.2 Nurse staffing levels and mix

The post-NHS reform creation of provider units ('trusts') established several hundred employing units who had greater 'freedom' and autonomy (in theory, at least) in determining nurse staffing levels and mix than had the pre-reform DHAs and Boards.

In the new market for health care, provider's income no longer derived directly from central budgets but from purchasers choosing to contract for their services. The key requirement for management in provider units was to achieve reductions in their costs, so that they remained competitive. The importance of labour costs (which are three-quarters of total cost) focused attention on staffing levels, skill mix and unit labour costs. Nursing, which represented the majority of direct care staff in most units, therefore came under cost-based scrutiny. The new Labour government of 1997 is continued to focus on cost containment, signalled that it anticipated trust mergers, but also highlighted the end of the 'internal market'. Policy emphasis is now on collaboration and integrating services.

In relation to nurse staffing levels and staffing mix at local level, the effect of the reforms were less about dismantling bureaucracy than about stimulating local management to review custom and practice and historical staffing patterns, with a view to achieving better 'value for money'. In this context there was continuing tension between those nurses and other health care professionals focusing on patient care, and those managers responsible for cost-effective use of resources but constrained by a lack of clinical knowledge. In combative language, this has sometimes been characterised by managers as 'taking on the professions', or ending 'professional tribalism'. It is unlikely that the change in government in 1997, or changes in policies will defuse this situation.

This combative stance was most evident in the immediate post reform period. It has since been tempered by realism, on the part of some managers, and also by a lack of resources to underpin radical changes in staffing. Many employing units have instigated skill-mix reviews or are attempting to re-profile their nursing workforce. These reviews are often linked to the introduction of support workers or vocationally qualified Health Care Assistants (HCAs). However, few trusts have secured a radical change in the workforce profile. Other areas where skill mix and role changes have been impacting on the nursing workforce are in the introduction of advanced clinical roles, the introduction of nurse practitioners, and in the changing deployment of enrolled nurses.

The 're-engineering' of some hospitals and implementation of 'patient focused care' practices, including the introduction of multi-skilled workers, also presents new challenges to the established health care professions. These challenges have continued under the Labour government, along with the likelihood of trust mergers. There has been continuing debate about the impact on the quality of care provided by some of the skill mix changes which are occurring in the NHS and little evidence that the majority of these changes have been subject to any evaluation (see Buchan, Seccombe, Ball, 1996). Evaluation of organisational characteristics, staff profile and outcomes, which has begun to be undertaken in so called 'magnet' hospitals in the United States (Aiken, Smith and Lake, 1994), has not yet been addressed in the UK.

In the absence of agreed and robust outcome measures, decisions on staffing mix are often being based primarily on considerations of cost. There has been little attempt to conduct a proper evaluation of the cost-effectiveness of skill-mix changes. Whilst short-term cost savings, in terms of a reduced paybill can be achieved, little attention has been paid to evaluating the broader impact on cost and quality in terms of employee productivity and effectiveness of care provided (Buchan and Ball, 1991). Some research suggests that there is a direct relationship between the grade mix of nursing staff used and measures of the quality of care, with a 'richer' skill mix leading to higher quality of care (Carr-Hill *et al*, 1992).

Whilst there are cost-based factors pushing managers to consider 'cheaper' staff mixes, one possible constraint on further developments towards a less skilled or qualified, but 'cheaper' NHS nursing workforce, could be the parallel drive towards lowering costs of patient care by reducing the average length of patient stay. The achievement of higher patient throughput, with a higher average acuity level, may place a limit on such skill mix changes, as there will be a continued requirement for highly skilled staff to treat high dependency patients.

These staffing changes have been occurring against a backdrop of continued increase in the workload of nurses in the NHS as provider units have attempted to increase productivity and reduce unit costs. Latest data from the NHS in England show that between 1990/91 and 1995/96 (Department of Health, 1996a):

- the total number of ordinary admission episodes rose by 11.4 per cent from 7.52 million to 8.38 million;

- total outpatient attendances increased by 11 per cent from 36.1 million to 40.1 million; and

- the number of day cases rose by over 100 per cent from 1.26 million to 2.85 million.

Against this background of increased activity it is difficult to assess the reform-led impact of changes in staffing patterns and levels, both in terms of changes in employee numbers and in terms of their effect on the level of costs and quality of service being provided. Change is incremental, and varies in pace and in direction in different employing units.

1.3 Employee relations

The period up to and during the NHS reforms was also one in which the Conservative government had introduced various laws restricting the role of trade unions. Generally, the 1980s and early 1990s were a time of high unemployment, and constrained union power. This was symbolised by the growing use of 'human resource management' techniques in the NHS and other areas of the public sector (see Seccombe and Buchan, 1994).

Employee relations in the pre-reform NHS were heavily unionised, with policy and procedure determined nationally but interpreted and applied locally. As with much else in the public sector, the employee relations system in the NHS was a post-war development of the welfare state, with national negotiating committees (Whitley Councils) being established for the various staff groups.

The Whitley system of national Councils comprised management and union representatives. These were little changed from the inception of the NHS in 1948 until the implementation of the reforms in the 1990s. Often characterised as unwieldy, unresponsive and overly bureaucratic, the Whitley Council system has been a major target for criticism (see, for example, McCarthy, 1976).

The whole thrust of the NHS reforms, with their emphasis on local management's right and responsibility to manage, the anti-bureaucratic language, and the 'freedom' given to self-governing trusts to establish local employee relations machinery, reflected political and managerial frustration with the lack of national political control and limitations on local managerial influence over the Whitley system.

Whitley is an easy target for criticism and jibes about bureaucracy, yet the implementation of the NHS reforms saw no rapid move away from its sphere of influence. This was perhaps unsurprising, given some of the checks incorporated in the NHS Act (for example, NHS employees whose workplaces become self-governing trusts had the right to remain on Whitley terms and conditions), but also reflected a pragmatism at local level which was not required of national level politicians and civil servants. If the influence of Whitleyism was to be reduced, or ended, some alternative system for employee relations would have to be in place, which was capable of supporting productive management-staff relations locally and nationally.

In an organisation where centralised negotiations have been institutionalised, and where there has previously been less need to develop a full range of local level negotiating skills, such changes could not happen overnight - even if all the parties involved were to regard such developments as desirable. Initial opposition to such developments from trade unions, and a 'wait and see' approach by some managers prior to the results of the 1992 General Election, in which the opposition Labour Party were committed to reversing some elements of the reform programme, also acted to slow the initial pace of change. In practice, the Whitley Councils survived largely intact the period of Conservative government. Ironically, it is the election of a Labour government in 1997 which may lead to significant changes. At the time of writing there is increased pressure from employers represented by the NHS Confederation, and by some unions (*eg* UNISON) to review the operations of Whitley.

The main effort of local management activity in employee relations since the NHS reforms was directed at simplifying the processes and procedures involved. This activity was mainly directed at establishing 'single table' recognition agreements, where all employee relations activity is conducted in one forum, with a limited number of union representatives (in some cases full time officials being excluded or having observer status only). It has largely been left to the unions to decide which of their representatives will sit at the 'table'. Where this has occurred, it was often the small specialist professional associations who lost out.

Most local managers have tended to adopt a pragmatic and long-term approach, rather than going for radical short-term change. New recognition agreements tend, therefore, to reflect Whitley in terms of the number of staff groups recognised. This reflects most managers' pragmatism in adopting an incremental approach. This can more flexibly respond to changes in the political and labour market climates and can be altered when circumstances dictate. Reporting on plans for change in employee relations for nurses, at the time of the reforms, Buchan (1992) noted that:

'No trust or directly managed unit is a green field site on which a new industrial relations culture and pay determination process could be set up on

April 1st 1991. Organisational status may have changed on that date, but the organisational politics, personalities, industrial relations custom, practice and history remain.'

The end result of this pragmatism, trade union resistance, lack of resources and organisational inertia is that six years later, the majority of nurses remain linked to the Whitley system. It is likely that the new Labour government may exert some top-down changes in the Whitley system as part of a broader process of change in the climate of NHS employment relations, but that a national framework will be retained.

1.4 Nurses' pay

NHS nurses' pay has, since 1983, been determined by an independent Review Body, which takes annual evidence from nursing unions and organisations, and from management. It then makes recommendations on pay increases. National Whitley meetings continue to cover other aspects of employment.

The NHS reforms of the late 1980s raised the prospect of a fundamental move away from this centralised approach to determining nurses' pay. This was a result both of the setting up of self-governing trusts, and because the focus on labour costs stimulated by the purchaser/ provider split was bound to increase demands from local management to have greater control of paybill size and allocation. Further stimulus came from the Citizens' Charter, which emphasised the need for the pay of NHS employees and other public service workers to be more closely linked to local performance. The pressure was to move from national to locally determined pay.

As with NHS employee relations systems in general, the post reform pace of change in the ways that NHS nurses' pay was determined was probably slower than those responsible for the reforms would have envisaged or would have desired.

Whilst there has been much trust level activity in creating job evaluation systems, training staff in pay negotiation skills, and attending conferences and seminars on local pay, there have been comparatively few examples of this activity becoming fully operationalised. Most trusts continue to pay most, or all, nurses on Review Body rates, and employ them on associated Whitley terms of employment. The Review Body made recommendations in 1995 and 1996 which included a local pay element (see Chapter 4 for details), but in 1997 reversed this practice. Whilst they remain committed in principle to some element of local pay, the Review Body noted in their 1997 report that *'There has been little effective use made of local pay in respect of the vast majority of nursing staff who remain on Whitley or shadow Whitley contracts'*, (para 27). They also noted that *'Trusts have generally failed to take the initiative in the development of their local pay strategies . . .'*, (para 24); and that those trusts that have been attempting to introduce change have been hampered by *'an absence of funds . . . and the right of staff to retain their Whitley contracts'*, (para 29). The new Labour government appears committed to retaining a national framework of 'core' pay and conditions, but may permit local 'flexibility'.

The Labour government, elected in 1997, is less enthusiastic about 'full blown' local pay, but is equally unlikely to turn back the clock on NHS pay determination. Local 'flexibility' is likely to be supported, within a framework which reflects concerns for improving the position of low paid staff, and for supporting equal pay for equal worth.

Some recent developments have been stimulated, and others hindered, by management concern about equal pay legislation. Much of the activity on job evaluation, for example, reflects attempts by NHS trusts to establish 'defensive' systems to prevent any equal pay claims. In April 1997 the Department of Health settled two of the 18 test cases brought under the 'equal pay for work of equal value' changes to the Equal Pay Act[3]. The so-called Enderby case involved a speech therapist who, in 1986, launched a claim for pay parity with clinical psychologists (the act had previously covered only cases in which women could show that a man doing the same, or broadly similar, work, was being paid more). Some 1,500 other speech therapists have lodged claims and the case is likely to encourage other 'female' occupations, including nurses and midwives to follow.

The proposed and actual changes to the way in which NHS nurses' pay is determined raise important questions about the likely impact on labour market behaviour. These issues will be examined in Chapter 5.

1.5 Nursing education

Nursing education has gone through a period of considerable change with the implementation of Project 2000 and the introduction of the internal market to education. Project 2000 was introduced in phases in England beginning in 1989, and implemented in Scotland and Wales in 1992. As part of Project 2000, the traditional three year courses leading to first level registration (registered nurse) were phased out, while two-year courses leading to second level registration (enrolled nurse) were discontinued.

The new pre-registration diploma programme was developed in response to changes in health care policy, in particular, the shift in health care policy towards greater provision in the community and increased emphasis on health promotion. It was also a response to the forecast reductions in the pool of traditional entrants (*ie* school leavers) to nurse education.

In addition to changes in content, pre-registration diploma nursing courses differ from traditional courses in several important respects. Diploma students are college based and supernumerary for most of their clinical placements in hospitals and the community. They make a lower rostered service contribution (of about 20 per cent) to patient care, mainly in the later stages of their course. The full implications for workforce planning of these fundamental changes in nurse education have not always been fully appreciated.

1.6 Nursing 'shortages'

The existence of a match, or mismatch, between supply and demand determines the existence and size of a 'shortage' or oversupply of nurses. Nursing shortages have been a recurring theme in NHS nursing and in other countries. Less frequently, temporary oversupply of 'new' nurses coming from pre-registration education has been a problem. Either situation creates organisational difficulties, is usually given a high profile by the media, and is an embarrassment for the government of the day.

In examining issues of shortage and oversupply, one key point to highlight is the notion of *willingness* on the part of the potential nurse to enter the labour market, and on the part of the employer to pay the 'going rate'. A 'shortage' is not merely about a numbers game, it is about individual and collective decision-making and choice.

Another factor which has to be stressed is the time-lag between decisions which determine the number of potential 'new' nurses entering pre-registration education, and those nurses entering the labour market as qualified practitioners. This lag of four to five years is built into the commissioning system for nursing education. Employers 'signal' their likely future requirement for nurses, and this indicator, at aggregate level, is used along with other information (retirement rates, turnover rates *etc.*) to inform decision on the size of future intakes into pre-registration education. The process is complicated by the need to estimate future demand for nurses from non-NHS employers (independent hospitals, nursing homes *etc.*).

Shortages of qualified nursing staff have increasingly been highlighted in the media since 1995. However, there has been a marked disagreement between interested parties as to their nature and extent. Much of this debate about nursing shortages has been conducted in the context of the pay determination process and this places major constraints on determining an objective viewpoint.

There is unanimity amongst the various parties regarding the existence of localised shortages in particular specialties and also agreement that much evidence is anecdotal. In their written evidence to the Review Body the Departments of Health have repeatedly denied that there is a national shortage (although admitting to increasing supply problems); the Trust Federation and the National Association of Health Authorities and Trusts (now the combined NHS Confederation) promoted the idea of regional shortages (rather than local); and the unions have argued that there are widespread problems requiring national solutions.

The Review Body, in its 1997 report, are of the view that signs of a general shortage may be emerging. They also highlight that higher workloads, combined with vacancies, can have a marked impact on trusts' ability to provide services (para 95).

A 'national' shortage could be defined as occurring when *all* specialties report problems in *all* localities. If we accept this definition then clearly there is not currently a 'national' shortage, and probably never has been. A more appropriate definition of national shortage may be one in which there is agreement that there is a sufficient critical mass of specialty and geographically based staffing shortages to require nationally based monitoring and a nationally co-ordinated response. The erosion of relevant 'official' data in recent years is making this monitoring exercise more and more difficult. The Review Body has highlighted its concern about inadequate data and a lack of a strategic response to recruitment, and retention by the Department of Health and trusts.

The link between pay determination, recruitment and retention, has meant that in the past the Health Departments were unwilling to concede that there was such a 'national' shortage. This might reflect the fact that a central element of their argument in favour of local pay was that local problems required local solutions. This position was totally reversed, to the surprise of the Review Body, in 1997, with the Departments arguing that using local pay for this purpose could lead to wage spirals (para 96).

Away from the pay determination arena, there has been a greater willingness on the part of official bodies to acknowledge the uncertainties of nurse workforce planning, and the increasing potential for staffing problems. In an executive letter to the Chief Executives of all NHS trusts and Health Authorities, the Director of Human Resources of the NHS Executive highlighted the need for *'robust workforce planning'* in the education commissioning process for pre-registration nurse education (EL(95) 96, 23 August 1995). In an annex to this letter, Planning Guidance for education commissioning authorities was set out. This 'official' view highlighted concern about the likelihood of increasing staffing problems in the NHS and pinpointed the major factors acting to create these shortages. In contrast to the last cycle of nursing shortages which happened in the mid to late 1980s, and which was primarily due to increasing *demand* for healthcare and for staff, the current concern focuses both on *supply* and *demand* issues. In short, the *conditions* for nursing shortages are more pronounced now than they were two or three years ago, and official 'best guesses' suggest that these conditions will become even more evident over the next few years.

Nursing shortages have been a recurring focus of concern in the UK. There have been a number of 'official' reports published since the 1930s which have attempted to examine the reasons for shortages and to propose solutions (see Appendix 1 for details).

The Briggs Report, published almost 25 years ago, is the most recent national 'official' independent report to have acknowledged nursing shortages, examined causes in detail and highlighted potential solutions. Reports with a national focus published since then have been concerned primarily with supporting the need for changes in nurse education *(eg* the 'Judge' Commission), or have focused on broader policy change in relation to nursing (*eg* the Kings Fund Report *'New for Old'*, published in 1990). Other publications have tended to be based on surveys of individual nurses, *eg* (Price Waterhouse (1987), and the series of surveys commissioned by the RCN and conducted by the IES which are the basis of thus book). Others have been critiques of current management methods by quasi-governmental bodies (National Audit Office; Audit Commission). These studies have all made valuable contributions to the understanding of the dynamics of the nursing labour market and the motivation of individual nurses, but none has taken what could be termed a 'rounded' assessment of supply and demand issues. The aim of this book is to make a contribution to filling that gap.

1.7 Structure of the book

The rest of the book is structured in eight chapters:

Chapter 2 presents a profile of the current dimensions and dynamics of the UK nursing labour market.

Chapter 3 describes the working patterns, working hours and contracts of registered nurses.

Chapter 4 gives detailed consideration to turnover, 'wastage' and workloads.

Chapter 5 discusses nurses' pay and labour market behaviour, drawing on research from the UK and abroad.

Chapter 6 highlights the changing career patterns of nurses as the health sector is reformed and organisations are restructured.

Chapter 7 provides a critique of developments in the system of workforce planning in the UK nursing labour market, and highlights the main challenges to the system.

Chapter 8 discusses the likely future trends in the UK labour market for nurses, and presents the results of modelling of 'what if' scenarios.

Chapter 9 provides conclusions and an overview.

2 The UK Nursing Labour Market

2.1 Introduction

This chapter profiles the labour market for nurses in the UK. It provides an overview of the dimensions and dynamics of the labour market, and sets the scene for the more detailed examination in the late 1990s of labour market behaviour presented in subsequent chapters.

2.2 The dimensions of the nursing labour market

In March 1996 there were 645,011 qualified nurses, midwives and health visitors registered with the UK Central Council (UKCC) for Nursing, Midwifery and Health Visiting. This is the 'pool' from which the NHS, and other employers, must recruit qualified staff.

The 'pool' has grown year on year, until recently, when there was a small dip in 1993/94, followed by an upward adjustment the following year (see Table 2.1).

Table 2.1 The 'pool' of registered nurses, 1991 to 1996

Year	Number of nurses on UKCC effective register
1991	622,001
1992	633,119
1993	641,749
1994	638,361
1995	642,951
1996	645,011

Source: UKCC Statistical Analysis of the Council's Professional Register

2.2.1 Gender mix

Nine out of every ten nurses (91 per cent) on the Register are female, but there is evidence that the proportion of men in the profession is on the increase. Of the 645,011 practitioners on the UKCC Register 59,000 (9.2 per cent) were men. This represents about 6,600 more males on the Register than in March 1991, an increase of 11.2 per cent at a time when the overall Register had grown by only 3.6 per cent. Even in 1993-94, when the total number of registered practitioners declined for the first time in many years, the number and proportion of males on the Register increased.

The comparatively small numbers of practitioners on the Register who have come through the Project 2000 route, and the short timescale during which they have been registering (since 1993), limits useful interpretation of data on this group. But there is some indication that the implementation of Project 2000 has increased the proportion of men coming into the profession.

The growth in the numbers of men in nursing should not be overstated. In percentage terms, the increase has been from 8.5 per cent in 1990/91 to 9.2 per cent in 1995/96. Although this is a consistent upward trend, it is less significant in workforce planning terms than the overall decline in the size of 'new' intakes to the profession, and the ageing of the nursing workforce as a whole.

2.2.2 Ethnicity

Until recently, national data on the ethnic composition of the nursing workforce were not routinely collected. These data were first collected in the 1994 Non-Medical Workforce Census for England but were not published because they were regarded as unreliable. Data on ethnicity collected by the 1995 Non-Medical Workforce Census were released in May 1997. These data revealed that the majority of registered nurses are white (see Figure 2.1) (Department of Health, 1997).

The proportion of nurses who are black rose with age. For example, 5.6 per cent of those aged 45-54 and 8.7 per cent of those aged 55-64 were black compared with only 0.8 per cent of those aged under 25 and 2.2 per cent of those aged 25-34.

This pattern of a shrinking proportion of nurses coming from ethnic minorities is unlikely to change in the near future. According to the 1995 Non-Medical Workforce Census only 4.8 per cent of learners were black.

Figure 2.1 Ethnic origin of registered nurses in the NHS (England) as at September 30, 1996

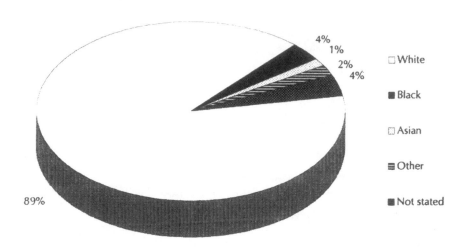

Source: Department of Health, 1997, *Statistical bulletin: NHS hospital and community health services non-medical staff in England: 30 September 1996*, Government Statistical Office

Data on entries to pre-registration diploma and degree programmes in 1996/97 (England) reveals that only 3.8 per cent of entrants were black.

These data highlight the comparative failure of the NHS to attract ethnic minority recruits to the nursing profession. Many of the black nurses recruited to the NHS in the 1960s were employed as enrolled nurses, and had limited career opportunities. Research (Beishon *et al*, 1995, Pudney and Shield 1997) has suggested that nurses from ethnic minorities continue to be discriminated against in their employment and their rate of career progression.

2.2.3 Age profile

One major shift in the profile of the profession is in its age distribution. The profession has 'aged' rapidly in recent years, mainly as a result of comparatively smaller intakes of new (and younger) practitioners from pre-registration education. In 1990/91, 26 per cent of all nurses on the Register were less than 30 years of age, by 1995/96 this age group had dropped to 17 per cent of the total (see Figure 2.2). The surveys conducted by the IES have recorded a similar shift in the nursing workforce. The average age of nurses covered by the annual surveys increased from 37 in 1986 to 40 in 1997. This ageing parallels trends in the United States where the average age of RNs in 1992 had increased to 43 years (Wunderlich *et al*, 1996).

Figure 2.2 Age profile of registered nurses, 1990 and 1996

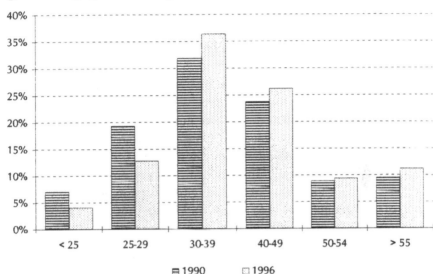

Source: UKCC Statistical analysis of the Council's Professional Register

A statistical 'bulge' of nurses in their mid-30s to mid-40s is working its way through the system, reflecting the large intakes to nurse education of the 1970s and early 1980s. As age is a major determinant of labour market behaviour, an 'ageing' workforce will have implications for planning, staff utilisation and priorities in reward strategy. The stereotyping of nurses as mobile, young and female, was never a true reflection of the profile of the profession but is increasingly becoming even more of a misrepresentation.

2.2.4 Student nurses

There were approximately 3,000 (wte) learner nurses and over 40,000 (headcount) pre-registration diploma students in the UK (at September 1996). Learners are nurses on traditional (*ie* pre-Project 2000) training courses. With the full implementation of Project 2000, today's student nurses are receiving college based education, and have supernumerary status during work experience, unlike those trained on 'traditional' courses.

A recent survey of 2,000 nursing students (Seccombe, Jackson and Patch, 1995) revealed that the profile of nursing students was changing in accordance with the aims of Project 2000. The proportion of men in the intakes had risen to 15 per cent of the most recent entrants. On average, nursing students were older than in the 1970s, with more than a third of respondents being aged over 25. A third of nursing students were married or living with partners and nearly a quarter had dependent children. The survey also showed an improvement in the educational background of entrants. The proportion of nursing students with A levels (or equivalents) had doubled since the 1970s. Finally, a high proportion of nursing students were shown to have had quite considerable work experience before coming into nursing, and for many that experience was in the health care sector.

One of the key determinants of future nurse supply is the level of drop-outs from pre-registration education. Wastage from training varies by region and by cohort (Seccombe, Jackson and Patch, 1995) and it is not easy to reconcile intake and drop-out figures as presently collected. There is no consensus on the drop-out rate. Figures for England show that the number of discontinuations was equal to 11 per cent of entrants to pre-registration courses in 1995/96 or 5 per cent of the in-training population as at the end of March 1996 (ENB, 1997). Data for Scotland (Scottish Office, 1997) show that the proportions of the 1992/93 intakes to diploma courses who failed to complete, ranged from 20.9 per cent on the Adult branch to 35.1 per cent on Paediatrics. Meanwhile wastage rates for successive cohorts have fallen. For example, wastage from the first year of the Adult branch programme reduced from 10.1 per cent in 1992/93 to 8.6 per cent in 1994/95. Figures for Northern Ireland show that the number of discontinuations were equal to 2.7 per cent of the in-training population at the end of March 1996 compared to 3 per cent in March 1996 (National Board for Northern Ireland 1996). Evidence suggests that around 15 per cent of those who embark on pre-registration nursing courses do not complete them. In addition a small proportion of those who qualify and are eligible to register, do not do so. When determining education and training places, commissioners need to make sufficient allowance for such wastage.

2.2.5 Nurses in paid employment

The main employer recruiting from the 'pool' of nurses on the UKCC register is the NHS, which employs approximately half of all nurses on the Register. A detailed picture of the number of qualified nurses in other forms of employment is difficult to establish, because of the fragmented nature of the employer base. Table 2.2 gives estimates for the major employers. Nurses are also employed in other sectors. For example, 3,350 nurses have recorded an occupational health nursing qualification (UKCC, 1996) and there are more than 6,000 Marie Curie nurses in the UK, of whom approximately two-thirds are registered nurses (*Directory of Hospice and Palliative Care Services in the UK and Republic of Ireland, 1996*). Others are employed in the armed forces, the prison service, the voluntary sector, *etc.*

Table 2.2 Number (wte) of registered nurses employed in nursing, by sector, 1995

1. NHS (UK)	305,160 wte
2. Independent Acute/Nursing Homes (GB)	57,775 wte
3. GP practice nursing (GB)	10,478 wte

Source: Department of Health Statistical Bulletin/ Department of Health Annual Return KO36: Private Hospitals, Homes and Clinics registered under Section 23 of the Register Homes Act 1984/ Department of Health bi-annual census of general medical practitioners/ Scottish Health Statistics/ Welsh Office (Department of Health)/ Department of Health and Social Security, Northern Ireland

In overall terms, approximately four times as many nurses work in the NHS as in all other forms of nursing employment. However, in recent years, *net growth* in nursing employment has been accounted for by increased employment in the various non-NHS sectors. Whilst overall employment in the NHS has remained largely static since the late 1980s (see Figure 2.3), the number of nurses working in the independent sector has *tripled*, and the number of nurses working as practice nurses has *quadrupled*.

The growth of non-NHS employment for nurses is of significance, both because it explains the continued high participation rate of nurses in employment (see next section) and because it requires careful consideration when determining policy in relation to workforce planning and remuneration strategy for NHS nurses. Until recently, the NHS, as monopoly 'provider' of registered nurses, and near monopsony employer of nurses, did not give much consideration to the competitive position of the non-NHS sectors. These sectors recruit from the same pool of registered staff, but do not participate in the education of new entrants to the pool —

Figure 2.3   Change in number (wte) of registered nurses employed by the NHS, 1974 to 1995 (GB)

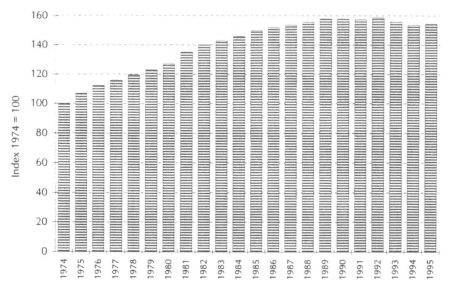

Source: Seccombe and Smith, 1997a

the NHS and public sector remain the only source of new entrants (with the exception of nurses coming to the UK from abroad) to the UKCC Register.

The 'monopsony effect' of the NHS in earlier decades has important implications for labour market behaviour and for nurses' pay. As the dominant employer, NHS pay rates have in the past dictated what the 'market rate' for nurses pay will be, rather than the 'market' dictating what NHS nurses pay should be. The move from a single national NHS rate to potentially varying local NHS pay rates, may complicate this situation. However, in economic terms, at both national and local level, the NHS is likely to continue to exert near monopsonistic power in purchasing the services of registered nurses - that is, it will usually be the major employer of nurses in a specific labour market.

The implementation of the NHS Act in April 1991 created a situation in which there were several hundred trusts, each acting as an employer. In many labour markets, the major competition for nurses is between NHS units, rather than with other, non-NHS employers. In particular, in larger conurbations and metropolitan areas, several trusts may be competitors in recruiting and retaining nurses. The labour market implications of this local 'competition' - real or apparent - are discussed in Chapter 5, which examines the impact of local pay.

2.3 Dynamics of the labour market

If the UKCC Register represents the pool, or potential 'stock' of nurses from which all employers must recruit, a number of 'flows' to and from the pool can be identified. These macro level flows highlight the extent to which the overall labour market for nurses is dynamic, with a continued inflow of new and 'returner' entrants, and a continued outflow of temporary and permanent leavers. Evidence from various sources (*eg* Lader, 1995 and unpublished health service data) consistently suggest that, at a national level, around three-quarters of those entering nursing employment do so from pre-registration education; the remainder enter employment from the pool or from overseas.

There are three sources of 'inflow', or new additions to the 'pool' of nurses on the UKCC Register. These are new entrants to the Register from education in the UK; re-entrants or 'returners' to nursing, and new entrants from non-UK sources.

2.3.1 New entrants

The number of new entrants from nurse education has begun to decline in recent years. Intakes to first level nursing courses fell from 19,600 in 1987/88, to 15,472 in 1995/96, and provision of second level courses (for enrolled nurse qualifications) has ended. The overall effect has been a reduction in intakes to pre-registration education of more than 7,500 (or 33 per cent) since the late 1980s (see Table 2.3).

The knock-on effect of these reductions in intakes to nurse education is beginning to show in the falling levels of initial entries to the UKCC Register. Table 2.4 shows that new entries, from the UK, fell by over 2,000 (11 per cent) between 1990/91 and 1995/96. Over this period, the numbers entering the Register from pre-registration education in Northern Ireland fell by 12 per cent, in Scotland by a quarter (24 per cent) and in Wales by 16 per cent.

2.3.2 Returners

The second source of inflow is qualified practitioners returning to paid nursing employment after a career break or time spent in other activities. These nurse 'returners' were one of the main subjects of scrutiny in the recently published survey (Lader, 1995) conducted by the Office of Population Censuses and Surveys (OPCS). This detailed study, based on

Table 2.3 Entries to pre-registration nursing courses 1987/88 to 1995/96, by country

	England		Scotland		Wales		N. Ireland		UK Total	
	Level 1	Level 2	Level 1	Level 2	Level 1	Level 2	Level 1	Level 2	Level 1	Level 2
1987/88	15,202	2.597	2,638	585	983	199	787	24	19,610	3,405
1988/89	15,905	1,682	2,734	529	892	135	854	1	21,221	2,347
1989/90	15,797	587	2,837	399	993	47	815	0	21,117	1,033
1990/91	15,452	62	2,779	204	1,010	74	697	0	20,676	340
1991/92	16,864	0	2,146	84	712	0	745	0	21,406	84
1992/93	15.921	0	2,348	55	945	0	642	0	20,694	55
1993/94	12,464	6	2,377	27	871	0	528	0	16,737	33
1994/95	10,844	0	2.230	9	705	0	466	0	14,245	9
1995/96	12,033	0	2,209	4	754	0	476	0	15,472	4

Source: Seccombe and Smith, 1996/ English National Board/ Welsh National Board/ National Board for Scotland/ National Board for Northern Ireland

Table 2.4 New entries to the UKCC Professional Register from the UK, 1990/91 to 1995/96

	1990/91	1991/92	1992/93	1993/94	1994/95	1995/96
England	14,786	14,184	13,931	13,992	13,997	13,527
N. Ireland	659	726	717	707	585	581
Scotland	2,537	2,513	2,485	2,334	2,060	1,920
Wales	998	846	936	915	769	842
Total	**18,980**	**18,269**	**18,069**	**17,948**	**17,411**	**16,870**

Source: Seccombe and Smith, 1997a

data from the 1991 census and a follow-up survey in 1993, considered the number of potential 'returners' to nursing, and discussed the measures required to encourage them back to nursing.

Improving the 'return rate' to nursing after career breaks has been a recurrent theme in workforce planning. As long ago as the 1930s, a report promoting solutions to nursing shortages highlighted the scope for attracting 'married nurses' back to work (Ministry of Health, 1939).

A previous study by the OPCS (Sadler and Whitworth, 1975) attempted to map out the dimensions and characteristics of the 'reserves' of potential returner nurses. This was based on census information and on follow-up interviews. Two-thirds of those not working in nursing at the time of the study (24 per cent of the total nursing population) were identified as 'intending to return to nursing' at some point.

Lader (1995) used similar methods and found a much smaller proportion of potential returners to nursing generally (not just returners to the NHS). This study reported that only one-third (32 per cent) of the sample of potential returners had returned, or intended to return to the profession.

Of the one-third of individuals with nursing qualifications in the 1990s who were not working in nursing, Lader reports that half were engaged in other types of employment (mainly in managerial 'white collar' and welfare-related jobs), leaving 15 per cent of the total population not in paid employment. Most of those 'non-working' individuals had worked in nursing, and cited domestic reasons and work dissatisfaction as their main reasons for leaving.

There is much agreement between different studies in terms of identifying factors likely to encourage return to nursing. Sadler and Whitworth (1975) reported the following factors as being most likely to encourage return: school holiday child care provision, crèche facilities, time off for child care, promoted posts for part-timers and better pay.

Similar results were found in a study of the Scottish nursing labour market (Waite *et al*, 1990). These findings were reinforced by Lader (1995) who found that refresher courses, greater availability of part-time work, more patient contact, 'return to nursing' opportunities, better resources, and training opportunities, were factors most likely to make a 'big difference' in encouraging the return of nurses to employment.

2.3.3 Non-UK entrants

The third source of inflows are entrants to the Register from non-UK sources - either nurses from abroad actively recruited by UK employers, or individuals moving to the UK who then enter the UK nursing labour market. Individuals with general first level nursing or midwifery qualifications from the other countries of the European Union (EU) can register with the UKCC via the European Community Directives for Nurses Responsible for Generic Care (77/452 + 77/453) and Midwives

(80/154 + 80/155); applicants from other countries have to apply to the UKCC for registration.

In practice, the UK appears to have diminished in importance in recent years as a destination for nurses who qualified in Australia and New Zealand, traditionally the main sources of overseas supply. Recently imposed restrictions on the granting of work permits to nurses (by the removal of nursing from its classification as a 'shortage' occupation) mean that entry from countries outside the EU is likely to be more difficult than in the past, although recent media attention has re-focused on UK hospitals recruiting abroad to address specialist skills shortages.

Applications to the UKCC for admission to the Register from nurses who qualified abroad have nearly halved since 1990/91, dropping to 4,218 in 1995/96. Admissions from overseas applicants to the UKCC Register have also fallen, by 13 per cent, in the same period. In overall terms, with the exception of Eire, overseas supply represents only a minor source of recruitment to UK nursing (for more detailed discussion on this subject, see Chapter 6 and see Buchan, Seccombe and Ball, 1992; Buchan, Seccombe and Thomas, 1997).

2.3.4 Outflows

Outflows from the pool may be temporary or permanent. Large numbers of nurses take one or more career breaks during their employment history, many with the firm intention of returning to paid nursing employment. Some of these nurses will maintain their registration, and be identified as part of the registered returner pool (the very fact that they maintain their registration may indicate their intention to return). Others will let their registration lapse, and will be taking a longer time out of nursing employment.

There has often been a tendency to characterise the totality of this outflow as 'wastage' from the profession, but it is clear that a proportion is voluntary and potentially temporary, whilst much of the rest is involuntary (statutory retirement, death, ill health). Reasons for the changing levels of turnover and 'wastage' are discussed further in Chapter 4. One key feature which merits specific policy attention is the impact of increasing levels of retirement amongst the nursing labour force, as the forthcoming 'retirement bulge' described in the previous section begins to take effect. The likelihood of increasing age related outflow from the profession occurring at a time when inflow from new registrants is falling and when the pool of returners may have reduced, will be explored in Chapter 8.

2.4 Participation rates and the non-nursing pool

There have been a number of attempts to combine official statistics and survey data to estimate participation rates and the size of the pool. This section reviews these past efforts and makes new estimates.

2.4.1 The 1971 Census

One of the earliest of these studies was undertaken by OPCS as part of the Briggs enquiry. This study used the 1971 Census to identify a sample of individuals (under age 52) living in Great Britain ' ... *who had nursing qualifications but who were not, at the time of the census, employed by the NHS as nurses'* (Sadler and Whitworth, 1975). Table 2.5 shows the number of female qualified nurses in each age group who were either working in NHS nursing, or not working in NHS nursing, and their estimated participation rates. Note that at this time participation was defined as working in NHS nursing.

Table 2.5 Best estimates of the number of 'qualified' nurses living in GB, 1971 (women)

	In NHS nursing	Not in NHS nursing	Total	Participation rate in NHS nursing
<25	33,530	13,480	47,010	71%
25-29	26,810	32,190	59,000	45%
30-39	43,290	52,710	96,000	45%
40-49	40,640	39,830	80,470	51%
50-70	40,750	78,660	119,410	34%
Total	**185,020**	**216,870**	**401,890**	**46%**

Source: Seccombe and Smith, 1997a/Sadler and Whitworth, 1975

This study showed a participation rate in NHS nursing of 46 per cent (women only) and an overall participation rate in nursing of 61 per cent. For men, the overall participation rate in NHS nursing was 70 per cent[4]. It is important to note that the definition of nursing was very broad. It simply meant that the interviewee had to indicate that they required a nursing qualification to obtain their job.

Of the overall pool of 105,000 nurses who were not nursing, approximately 65,000 (62 per cent) reported that they were likely to return to nursing at some point in the future, with two-thirds of these expecting to return within five years.

2.4.2 Survey-based estimates

Using survey data (n=2,325), Moores *et al* (1983) found an increase in participation rates in nursing for 'qualified' nurses, from 64 per cent in 1976 to about 70 per cent in 1980. A smaller survey (n=570) by Elias (1986) found a participation rate in nursing of only 51 per cent in 1984.

Waite *et al*, (1990) examined participation rates of registered nurses in Scotland using data from the 1981 Census and a sample survey of those who had qualified in Scotland between 1955 and 1985. The 1981 Census showed that 75 per cent of qualified nurses were in paid employment. Survey data for 1987 showed that participation in paid employment had risen to 85 per cent. The authors concluded that the rate of increase in participation by qualified nurses has been considerably faster than for the general female population as a whole.

A sample survey of individuals (n=14,332) holding second level registration with the UKCC in 1996 reported that 88 per cent of respondents were in paid employment (80 per cent in nursing employment and 8 per cent in non-nursing employment) (Seccombe, Smith, Buchan and Ball, 1997).

2.4.3 The Labour Force Survey

Wilson and Stilwell (1992) used data from the Labour Force Survey (LFS) to examine participation rates of those with nursing qualifications for the years 1983 to 1989. They identified an increase in the proportion of women with a nursing qualification who were employed in a nursing occupation from 51.5 per cent in 1983 to 57 per cent in 1989. The data for males showed a similar increase in participation, from 55 per cent in 1983 to 63.5 per cent in 1989. Overall participation, for men and women, increased from 52 per cent in 1983 to 57.5 per cent in 1989.

The approach used by Wilson and Stilwell can be applied to more recent data from the LFS (winter quarter, December 1996 to February 1997). According to LFS there were 734,278 individuals in the UK whose highest qualification was nursing: 610,640 (83.2 per cent) of these were in employment, 10,406 (1.4 per cent) were unemployed and 113,232 (15.4 per cent) were economically inactive. In the same quarter, there were 419,845 individuals employed as 'qualified' nurses which gives a participation rate in nursing employment of 69 per cent.

There are three main drawbacks with this approach. Firstly, the population is defined as those whose highest qualification was nursing, therefore it will exclude those who have other qualifications which they have self-reported as 'higher' than their nursing qualification. One-fifth (22 per cent) of those employed as 'qualified' nurses reported higher qualifications other than nursing, *eg* higher and first degrees, 'A' levels, NVQs, BTEC, teaching qualifications, *etc.* According to the LFS data the actual number of individuals employed in the winter quarter as 'qualified' nurses was 538,013 as opposed to 419,845.

Secondly, not all those (6.6 per cent) who reported that their highest qualification was nursing were employed as 'qualified' nurses, but worked as nursing auxiliaries, care assistants, nursery nurses or dental nurses.

Thirdly, having a nursing qualification is not the same as being on the UKCC Register, and therefore being eligible to work as a registered nurse.

One way of overcoming the first two of these issues is to recalculate the participation rate. Using the number of registered practitioners as the denominator gives a participation rate in nursing employment of 68 per cent for the UK. If we use the number of individuals employed as 'qualified' nurses as the numerator and the number of registered practitioners as the denominator then the participation rate in nursing employment rises to 87 per cent, which closely approximates some of the estimates reported in section 2.4.2.

2.4.4 The 1991 Census

The 1991 Census identified 454,880 people in England who were aged under 55 and who had qualified to be nurses, midwives or health visitors. Around 311,131 (68 per cent) of these worked in nursing, with 73,540 (16 per cent) working outside nursing and 70,030 (15 per cent) economically inactive.

These data are interesting for two further reasons. Firstly, the analysis reveals variations in the proportions who were working in nursing, in non-nursing employment or economically inactive, by region (Figure 2.4).

Within England, the proportion who had qualified as nurses and who were working in nursing ranged from 74 per cent in the North West to 64

Figure 2.4   Numbers working in or out of nursing, midwifery or health visiting, by standard region: 1991 Census

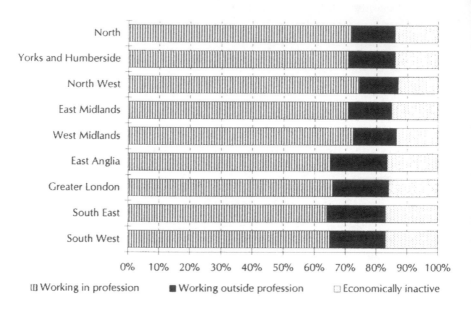

Source: Seccombe and Smith, 1997a/Lader, 1995

per cent in the South East. The economically inactive proportion ranged from 13 per cent in the North West and in the West Midlands, to 17 per cent in the South East and South West, and 16 per cent in Greater London. On this rather crude basis it would appear, somewhat paradoxically, that the potential pool was largest in those regions (London and the South East) which, anecdotally at least, were experiencing the greatest problems with recruitment.

Secondly, the census data illustrated an unexpectedly continuous decline in participation by age (Figure 2.5). According to these data, participation in nursing was at its highest (88 per cent) among those under 25, falling to 66 per cent at 35 to 39 and 64 per cent at 45 to 49. This contrasts with Sadler and Whitworth (1975) who found that participation in nursing was higher among those aged 40 to 49, than among those in their thirties or fifties. Equally, these data showed almost the same participation rates by age for both men and women.

Analysis from the 1991 LFS (England) showed a similar pattern of participation for individuals aged under 55 and whose highest qualification was nursing. According to the LFS there were 482,434 individuals whose highest qualification was nursing. At the same time there were 404,945 (86

Figure 2.5 Proportion working in nursing, midwifery or health visiting, by age: 1991 Census

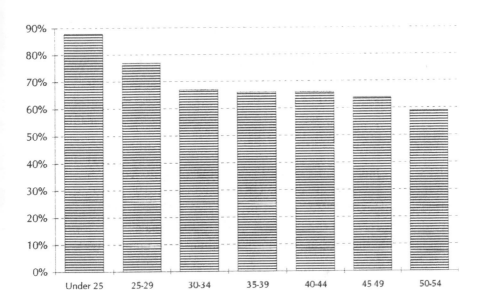

Source: Seccombe and Smith, 1997a/Lader, 1995

per cent) in paid employment, 66,118 economically inactive (14 per cent) and 11,370 unemployed (2 per cent). Further, there were 291,749 individuals working as 'qualified' nurses. This gives a participation rate of 72 per cent in nursing employment. The slightly higher participation rate in nursing employment, calculated from the LFS, may be due to differences in how people reported their highest qualification.

2.4.5 Why estimates vary

There are a number of reasons why participation rates in nursing may have been underestimated in the past, and consequently why the size of the non-nursing pool may be over-estimated. Most of these effects have been alluded to earlier. These reasons include the following:

• Individuals may have left nursing (*eg* because of ill-health, retirement or death) but remain on the Register until their next renewal date.

• Individuals on the Register may be living abroad.

- Individuals may maintain their UKCC registration because they regard it as relevant to their job, although they are not in, and are not available for, nursing employment. These would include health service managers, local authority managers, residential care home managers *etc.*

- Estimates based on the LFS or Census data (Sadler and Whitworth, 1975; Lader, 1995) refer to those holding nursing qualifications as the denominator. Whilst an individual may report having a nursing *qualification*, this is not necessarily the same as being on the UKCC Register.

This last point is illustrated in Table 2.6. It compares the age distribution of practitioners on the UKCC Register in 1991[5] with those who reported a nursing qualification at the time of the 1991 Census, and with those who reported that their highest qualification was nursing for the LFS. The Census and the LFS appear to overestimate the number of 'qualified' nurses. In the case of the LFS we know that a proportion of individuals whose highest qualification is nursing, work in occupations other than that of 'qualified' nurse.

Table 2.6 Age distribution of nurses, England, 1991: a comparison of three sources

	UKCC %	Census %	LFS %
<25	7.8	5.7	7.4
25–29	21.3	18.6	20.4
30–39	35.2	35.7	32.6
40–49	26.2	28.6	27.0
50–54	9.4	11.4	12.6
Total No.	*429,289*	*454,880*	*482,434*

Note: For comparative purposes this table excludes those aged 55 and over from the UKCC and LFS columns. Percentage figures in this and subsequent tables may not sum to 100 due to rounding

Source: Seccombe and Smith, 1997/ UKCC, Statistical Analysis of the Council's Professional Register/ Lader, 1995/ LFS, 1991

The OPCS study (Lader, 1995) excluded individuals aged over 55. In practice however, the Non-medical Workforce Census for 1991 (Department of Health, 1994) showed that 6.5 per cent of registered nurses in England, working in the NHS, were aged over 55. At the same time Atkin *et al* (1993) found that 22 per cent of all practice nurses in England were aged over 50. Data from the 1992 IES/RCN survey showed that 9 per cent of GP practice nurses and 9 per cent of nurses in the private sector were aged over 55 in 1991. Finally, the LFS showed that 5 per cent of individuals employed as 'qualified' nurses were aged over 55. Using the participation rate of 68 per cent and applying it to the whole population on the Register (including those aged over 55) leads to an overestimate of the pool because participation in nursing employment declines with age.

2.4.6 Estimating the 'pool' of returners

We conclude this section by providing new estimates of the number of registered nurses potentially available for nursing employment, *ie* the pool. A high proportion of nurses work part time; therefore, most nurse workforce data is presented as wte numbers. In order to gauge participation rates using the Register, the wte number has to be converted into a headcount figure. While the wte number for the NHS is based on a standard working week of 37.5 hours, there is no such standard for non-NHS employment.

We have estimated the wte for each nursing sector using official data sources for England. These figures were applied to data for the rest of the UK. We estimate that the minimum number of practitioners employed in nursing (UK) was 499,282 in 1995/96 (see Appendix 2 for derivations of the estimates). Using the number of practitioners (resident in the UK) on the Register as the denominator, participation in nursing employment is 81 per cent; this is similar to the 80 per cent found for second level registered nurses in 1996 (Seccombe, Smith, Buchan and Ball, 1997).

Not all practitioners on the Register are potentially available for nursing employment. Those over the age of 60 and resident in the UK represent 4.4 per cent of those on the Register. Further, a number of practitioners are employed in non-nursing work. Estimates of the proportion employed in non-nursing work range from 8 per cent (second level registered nurses) (Seccombe, Smith, Buchan and Ball, 1997) to 16 per cent (Lader, 1995). It is likely therefore that the pool of registered nurses, not in paid employment and aged under 60, is between 77,500 and 85,000. If we include those in non-nursing employment, the pool could be as big as 92,300. These figures are less the 140,000 qualified nurses which the Department of Health has estimated to be *'not working in nursing*[6].

The estimated pool is comparatively small and represents between 13 and 16 per cent of practitioners (see Figure 2.6) on the UKCC Register (aged under 60 and living in the UK). It is small relative to the number of vacant posts, implying that there are only five practitioners in the non-working pool for every vacancy. Of course, not all of those in the pool are able, or will want to, return to nursing. Given that the number of initial entries to the Register from training in the UK has fallen, due to smaller intakes to nurse education in the early 1990s, and that a substantial number of registrants are nearing retirement, the size of the pool is unlikely to grow over the short term. Furthermore, the number of returners from this pool may be comparatively small.

Figure 2.6 Nurses: in and out of work, 1997

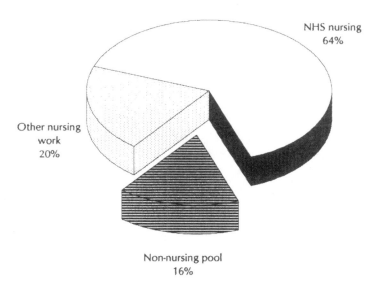

Source: Seccombe and Smith, 1997

2.4.7 Summary

The key features of the UK nursing labour market are an ageing, predominantly female workforce with a high participation rate in employment, sharply reduced new intakes, and a fragmenting employer base, as the NHS loses some of its monopsony power.

Key findings include:

- nine out of ten nurses are female; the proportion of them in nursing is growing, but from a low base;

- ethnic minority participation in nursing appears to have declined;

- the nursing workforce is ageing — the average age of nurses is now above 40;

- intakes to nurse education have declined rapidly, compared to earlier years;

- participation rates of nurses in paid employment have increased over the last two decades; and

- official estimates of the 'pool' of potential returners to nursing may be unrealistically high.

These features will have a major bearing on the future dynamics of the UK nursing labour market, and will be examined in detail in subsequent chapters.

3 Working Patterns and Employment Contracts

3.1 Introduction

The preceding chapter mapped key trends in the dimensions of the nursing workforce. Over the same period important aspects of nurse deployment, such as working hours and working patterns, have also changed. These are equally relevant in shaping the future of the nursing labour market. Indeed, the new Labour government has highlighted the need for 'flexible' employment in the NHS. This chapter describes the current working patterns, working hours and contracts of registered nurses, based on recent survey data.

It can be argued that working in full-time or part-time posts has been the traditional employment 'norm' for nurses in the UK labour market. The use of temporary nurses from a bank or agency has been the traditional source of additional 'flexibility' to cover for absence amongst permanent staff. Employing nurses on short-term contracts or longer fixed-term contracts has not been common procedure in the past, but evidence suggests that these are options which are increasingly being considered by NHS management and other employers as a reaction to the impact of the NHS reforms and changing labour market conditions.

In nursing in the NHS, the standard (*ie* 'normal') working week has been reduced considerably since the NHS was set up in 1948. This reduction, which occurred as a result of five separate changes in standard hours (see Figure 3.1) has cut the length of the working week by approximately one fifth over the last 50 years.

Such changes also have a direct impact on the nursing hours available to the NHS because reducing the standard hours worked effectively reduces the number of nursing hours available, unless additional overtime is worked, or more nurses are recruited. For example, the most recent reduction in standard hours, from 40 hours per week to 37½ hours per week in 1980, as part of the 'Clegg' (1980) package, equated to a 'loss' of

Figure 3.1 Standard working hours of NHS nurses

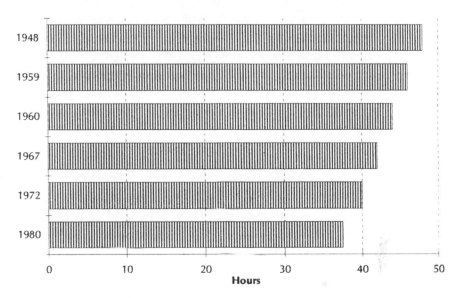

Source: Buchan, 1996

900,000 nursing hours, or 24,000 nursing and midwifery staff (at 37½ hours' whole time equivalent).

Each reduction in standard hours also had the effect of reducing, in aggregate form, the number of standard nursing hours available to the NHS. So any long-term assessment of trends in the supply of NHS nursing staff has to take account of changes in standard hours worked, if an accurate measure of the nursing hours available for patient care is to be determined.

3.2 Employment contracts

Conventionally, most nurses in employment have been employed on permanent employment contracts, with nurse bank and agency work being the 'traditional' temporary alternatives. However, mirroring general labour market changes, there has recently been an increase in the use of fixed-term contracts of employment.

NHS nurses working on a *fixed-term contract* basis cannot be identified separately using NHS data, so it is not possible to assess trends in use of such staff or to establish a national overview using official data. The 1996 IES/RCN survey found that 5 per cent of NHS nurses were employed on temporary (*eg* bank or agency) or fixed-term contracts (Seccombe and Smith, 1996). For the first time the IES/RCN survey was able to distinguish between those on temporary contracts and those on fixed-term contracts. Fixed-term contracts accounted for 70 per cent of respondents on non-permanent contracts. Furthermore, newly registered nurses were disproportionately represented among those on fixed-term or temporary contracts. By 1997, the proportion of NHS nurses on temporary contracts had declined to 3 per cent (Seccombe and Smith, 1997). (Note that temporary contracts excluded bank or agency contracts in the 1997 survey.) Data from the Independent Sector Workforce Survey suggest that 3.7 per cent of care and nursing staff in GB are employed on a temporary basis (Local Government Management Board, 1997).

In order to examine in more detail issues of contract based 'flexibility' in employment in NHS nursing, Buchan (1994b) conducted 12 case studies in NHS trusts. These case studies were undertaken in order to explore the rationales for changing working patterns.

The distribution of contract type is illustrated in Figure 3.2. Overall, the majority of qualified nurses in all the trusts were employed on permanent contracts, but there was a considerable variation between trusts

Figure 3.2   Contract status of qualified nurses (wte), by NHS trusts, September 1994

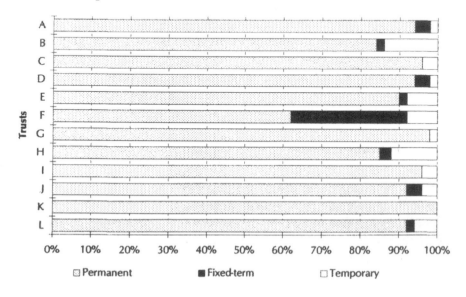

Note: Trusts A, B, C and D are teaching hospitals

Source: Buchan, 1994b

in the use of fixed-term and temporary contracts. For example, one in three (31 per cent) qualified nurses in trust F were employed on fixed-term contracts. Higher proportions (14 per cent) of qualified nurses employed on temporary contracts were found in trusts B and H, compared to other trusts.

Managers in the trusts cited several reasons for the use of *temporary* staff. These were uncertainty about future service levels, planned short term increases in workload (*eg* increased services funded by 'waiting list initiatives' money), cover for maternity leave, and the employment of newly qualified nurses awaiting permanent vacancies. With respect to the employment of bank nurses, some trusts reported that there was a reduction in the paybill (they are often employed on lowest increment, and usually do not receive pension payments or leave entitlement). The main reasons cited for the use of *fixed-term contracts* included using these staff to improve long-term flexibility of deployment, and uncertainty about future contracts and levels of service provision required.

The response from these trusts suggested that fixed term contract employment for qualified nurses was on the increase and was set to grow further. It also appears that much of the growth was a reflection of trusts entering the unknown of the 'managed market' and arose from uncertainties about the outcome of strategic reviews, rather than as a deliberate move towards a 'core periphery' model of employment (see Atkinson and Meager, 1986: ACAS, 1987) as a response to service contracts.

Data from the 1997 IES/RCN survey shows that 3 per cent of nurse respondents were employed on a *temporary* basis as agency or bank nurses (Seccombe and Smith, 1996). This is similar to the figure of 3 per cent quoted in response to a parliamentary question about the proportion of staff employed in the NHS as bank or agency nurses[7]. Analysis of previous years' data (Buchan, 1994b) has revealed wide regional variations in the extent of use of such staff, with fluctuating employment of agency staff, but an overall marked increase in the use of bank nurses in recent years.

Furthermore, Seccombe and Smith (1997) show that the proportion of NHS nurses who reported working on the bank, in addition to their main job, had increased from 29 per cent in 1991 to 56 per cent in 1997. The average number of hours worked each week by these NHS nurses on nurse banks had also risen, from 9 hours in 1991 to 11 hours in 1997.

3.3 Working patterns

Part-time working has been a traditional way of working for nurses. The provision of opportunities for part-time working, to improve recruitment and retention, has been a recurring theme in nursing for many years (see *eg* Auld (1967). Arguments for improved provision of part-time opportunities even pre-date the establishment of the NHS (Ministry of Health, 1947).

Survey data show that the incidence of part-time working has increased significantly over the last decade. For example data from the 1997 IES/RCN survey (Seccombe and Smith 1997) showed that nearly two-fifths (37 per cent) of all respondents employed in nursing were working part time compared with 27 per cent in 1987 (Waite *et al*, 1989). There was some variation between NHS and non-NHS nurses in terms of part-time working (33 and 37 per cent respectively).

The number of weekly contracted hours worked by part-time nurses varied across the three main employment sectors, with part-time NHS nurses contracted to work slightly more hours. Table 3.1 shows the average (mean) weekly contracted hours (and the standard deviation) worked by part-time nurses in the 1997 IES/RCN survey.

Table 3.1 Average weekly contracted hours for part-time nurses, by employment sector

	Contracted hours		
	mean	(sd)	Base no.
NHS nursing	23.5	(6.0)	862
Non-NHS nursing	21.9	(7.5)	168
GP practice nursing	20.3	(5.8)	197
All nurse respondents	22.8	(6.3)	1,227

Source: Seccombe and Smith, 1997a

The other main aspect of flexibility can be termed 'time based' flexibility and relates to different shift patterns and ways of deploying NHS nurses. There is a paucity of official data to provide any overview of the shift patterns being worked in NHS nursing. Survey based evidence *(eg* Seccombe and Smith, 1997) suggests that flexible shifts with a permanent night shift is the most common pattern of working for NHS nurses (see also Barton *et al*, 1993; Buchan, 1994b).

Data from the 1997 IES/RCN survey shows that nearly half of NHS nurses and non-NHS nurses (47 and 49 per cent respectively) worked shift patterns involving a mix either of earlies and lates, or earlies, lates and nights (see Table 3.2).

Table 3.2 Main work patterns by employment sector

Employment sector	Work Patterns (%)					
	Shifts Earlies/ Lates/ Nights	Shifts Earlies/ Lates	Days only	Permanent nights	Other	Base No.
NHS nursing	29	18	33	10	10	2,844
Non-NHS nursing	14	35	24	18	9	497
GP practice nursing	–	24	60	–	16	253
Bank/Agency nursing	22	32	20	13	13	151

Source: Seccombe and Smith, 1997a

There has been a trend towards greater devolution of responsibility for management decisions on patterns of shift working, with line managers and ward sisters in some trusts taking on responsibility to consult with their staff and decide what pattern of working is appropriate to their circumstances. Accompanying this trend is increased flexibility in deciding the 'start' and 'finish' times of shifts.

Previous research (Barton *et al*, 1993) has suggested that flexible shifts with a permanent night shift were most common in the NHS but that there was evidence to suggest a move towards more use of internal rotation, a reduction in fixed night shift working and more variation in the duration of shifts worked.

The cost of the unsociable hours payments made to NHS nurses working on shifts ('special duty payments') have been highlighted by management in evidence to the Review Body and were regarded by some commentators as a source of 'inflexibility' and a major area for action in relation to pay bill control when pay determination was localised (North West Thames RHA, 1992). In the mid 1990s some NHS trusts attempted to reduce the unsociable hours premia paid to nurses employed on trust contracts, and others tried to 'buy out' shift premia as part of establishing local pay and conditions (Incomes Data Services, 1994).

Despite this pressure the Review Body has not reduced special duty payments for a number of years. Other commentators have argued that to reduce or remove unsocial hours payments could introduce new 'inflexibilities', if nurses were then less willing to work unattractive hours. Results from the 1994 IES/RCN survey of nurses (Seccombe, Patch and Stock 1994) appeared to support this argument, as two-thirds of NHS nurses who were in receipt of unsocial hours payments reported that these payments were 'very important' in getting them to work unsocial hours.

Decentralised decisions on shift patterns and flexitime have previously been reported in some British hospitals (O'Byrne, 1989) but their use is more prevalent in nursing in the United States. In the US the use of flexitime in nursing has been cited as a factor in reducing dependency on agency staff and in increasing staff retention (Dison *et al*, 1981). Some US hospitals have taken this further and have established 'self scheduling', which in essence gives ward based nurses the freedom - and responsibility - to determine their own shift patterns, in agreement with the line manager. Self scheduling is now in use in a few NHS trusts (Buchan, Seccombe, and Ball, 1996).

Self scheduling is promoted in the US as an element in establishing a 'professional practice' model of nursing deployment and clinical autonomy (self governance). Various local studies have reported that its introduction has been linked to reduced turnover of nurses (Choi *et al*, 1986) and reduced time spent by managers in arranging work schedules (Miller, 1984). Some commentators in the US have also explicitly linked the introduction of this localised autonomy in decisions on working patterns with the expansion of 10- or 12-hour shifts. Miller (1984) noted that *'once staff nurses have control over their schedule, they may want to take the process a step further and institute combinations of 8, 10 and 12 hours shifts'*(p.35).

The 'pro' and 'anti' debate in relation to the use of 12 hour shifts in nursing has been continuing for many years in Britain, in the United States (see *eg* Jones and Brown, 1986; Fields and Loveridge, 1988; Palmer, 1991) in Australia (Bacon and Kun, 1986) and in New Zealand (O'Connor, 1992).

Many of the research studies based on a comparison of 8 and 12 hours shifts have only limited relevance, because they are usually localised, based on small sample sizes, often report on voluntarily accepted 12 hour shifts (rather than imposed changes in working patterns) and are also often written by the manager responsible for introducing them.

A further limitation is that the basis for evaluation and comparison is usually staffing indicators (turnover, absence, 'job satisfaction') or staff perceptions of quality of care, rather than independent assessment of the quality of care, levels of productivity and outcome under eight and 12-hour regimes. With all these caveats to ignore, it is not difficult to make a case 'for' or 'against' 12-hour shifts by selective use of the many small scale research publications which are available.

In a UK context, the series of research studies which best allow an examination which recognises and to an extent overcomes these limitations is that conducted by Reid and her colleagues. A study of the quality of care on ten wards found that nurses working a 12 hour shift scored lower on quality in planning, non physical care and evaluation of care, and that quality of care overall was 'significantly poorer' under a 12-hour shift regime (Todd, Reid and Robinson, 1989). Another paper, (Reid, Todd and Robinson, 1991) found lower levels of educational activity on 12-hour shifts. A study focusing on the quantity of nursing care provided on eight and 12-hour shifts found evidence of a 'pacing effect' on wards working to a 12-hour regime, with nurses taking more unofficial breaks, and comparative reductions in direct patient care (Reid, Robinson and Todd, 1993). Most recently, a survey of the views of nursing students and their tutors in relation to 12-hour shifts found students in favour but for 'social rather than professional reasons' and their educators very negative about the use of 12-hour shifts (Reid, Robinson and Todd, 1994).

On the basis of the available evidence it is not possible to be unreservedly pro- or anti- the use of 12-hour shifts but is important to recognise that the balance of the limited UK research available suggests that there can be negative aspects for patient care if nurses work 12-hour shifts. More generally, and again on the basis of available evidence, it can be suggested that some of these negative aspects may be more prominent if 12-hour shifts are imposed on reluctant staff rather than accepted voluntarily.

Another issue which appeared to be exciting increasing interest in a number of the trusts was the use of annualised hours - a system whereby employees are contracted to work an agreed number of hours in the year, but the actual number of hours worked per week are varied to match workload. Annualised hours are used in a number of industries (Incomes Data Services 1993) and their use has been cited as a means of effective deployment of groups of NHS staff working on a 24 hour basis (Mower and Rogers, 1993). Their use in NHS nursing has previously been reported in one NHS trust (see Incomes Data Services 1993; Buchan, 1994b).

In general terms, it has to be recognised that changes in working patterns which have evolved in the 1990s have done so against a backdrop of economic recession and high unemployment early in the decade. If labour market conditions and labour market behaviour change in the late 1990s and into the next century (*eg* if the trend in nurse turnover continues to increase from the lower level of the early 1990s, and skill shortages become more pronounced) so will the priorities and motivations of employers and employees.

In relation to the flexibility of deployment, there appears to be one fundamental issue still to be resolved. What would the impact be of any changes in deployment on cost-effectiveness and the quality of patient care? Independent evaluation of new working patterns (be it a revised shift pattern, or an increased use of temporary staff) is rarely undertaken, and even more rarely published. There are few published examples of detailed cost benefit analysis of alternative shift patterns, or of different configurations of 'core' and 'peripheral' staff in nursing. It is clear from the studies and data reviewed above that cost containment and the uncertainties of future service provision are at least as important in stimulating the introduction of new patterns of working as is a desire to improve patient care.

3.4 Summary

There has been an increase in recent years in the number of nurses working on short term fixed contracts, and nurses working temporarily on NHS banks:

- approximately two-fifths of nurses work part-time in their main jobs;

- 6 per cent of nurses in 1997 were working mainly on temporary contracts, or as bank or agency nurses; and

- the majority of nurses working in the NHS and elsewhere work some form of shift pattern - a three shift mix of 'earlies/lates' and nights being most common.

4 Turnover and Wastage

4.1 Introduction

Nurse retention and turnover were widely acknowledged as key concerns of health sector employers in the 1980s. At that time, NHS managers who had been traditionally dependent on a high proportion of school leavers entering nurse education felt exposed by projections of falling numbers of school leavers at a time of rising demand (Conroy & Stidston, 1988). To some extent the healthcare sector benefited from the recession of the late 1980s and early 1990s which took pressure off recruitment and retention. Comparatively high interest rates and mortgage costs, rising unemployment, and uncertain employment among nurses' spouses/partners contributed to the dampening down of turnover and job moves within nursing.

This recession effect has now dissipated. Vacancy rates for some groups are rising and retention is again a key issue for many employers of nurses.

4.2 Defining turnover and wastage

Turnover costs can also be a significant burden in terms of the direct and indirect use of resources. High rates of turnover may destabilise work groups through the loss of experienced staff, may have an adverse effect on staff morale, and may ultimately undermine the volume, continuity and quality of patient care (Audit Commission, 1997). Seccombe and Buchan (1991) identified average turnover costs of £3,000 when a NHS hospital replaced a leaving E grade staff nurse. Using the same methodology, a more recent study puts the average turnover costs at £4,900 (Audit Commission, 1997).

It is also important to recognise that there are benefits from a certain level of turnover. Most notably these benefits include: freeing up posts to allow new blood into the organisation; enabling career progression; providing opportunities for cost reduction.

Mapping and interpreting the level, characteristics, trends, and changing rationale for job changes within the nursing labour market, and flows into and out of this market, are important for several reasons. These include:

- turnover and wastage are key variables in determining the supply of registered nurses and in setting the number of nurse education places to be commissioned;

- an increasing level of job change within a sector may be an early warning of supply side problems; and

- turnover intentions are widely regarded as a good general barometer of job satisfaction.

The measurement of staff flows is difficult in the NHS. In particular, the lack of reliable and consistent information on the turnover and wastage of the nursing workforce is a continuing problem. In its Ninth Report on Nursing Staff, Midwives and Health Visitors (1992), the Review Body commented: *'We ... regret that reliable information on wastage from the NHS is not available'* (para. 42). Since then the available data set has probably deteriorated rather than improved. Indeed, in its 1997 report, the Review Body comments ' ... *we are left wondering how some Trusts can recruit, retain and motivate staff without adequate manpower data ...* ' (para. 100).

In this book we make the important distinction between turnover and wastage. Many studies use the term 'wastage' to mean all leavers. Here it is used only to refer to those leaving an employment sector (*eg* NHS nursing). The term 'turnover' is used to refer to the totality of leavers — which includes those moving within a sector (*eg* from one NHS trust to another), those moving between sectors (*eg* from NHS to non-NHS nursing) and those leaving paid employment altogether (*eg* to retirement).

It is important to have reliable data on both turnover and wastage, since the effectiveness of policies on recruitment, retention and the likelihood of return depend, in part, on knowing where leavers are going. The likelihood of a leaver returning is related to whether they leave the local labour market, whether they leave to raise a family, or whether they move to another NHS post. Lader (1995) shows that almost two-thirds of those who were out-of-service at the time of the 1991 census had returned to the profession as a registered nurse within two years.

For the NHS in England there were, until recently, limited data available centrally from the KM48 return, collated by the NHS Executive.

KM48 recorded information about numbers and whole-time equivalents of non-medical staff joining and leaving NHS trusts and Directly Managed Units. There were a number of important exclusions from KM48 (*eg* staff whose employment is of a casual or temporary nature) and it was widely regarded as inaccurate, incomplete and unreliable.

The KM48 data indicate an increase in wastage from NHS nursing in England during the early 1990s (Table 4.1). Just over 9 per cent of first-level, and 10 per cent of second-level registered nurses, left in 1994/95 — the last period for which these data were published.

Table 4.1 Registered nurses leaving the NHS: England

	Registered nurses, district nurses and health visitors	**Enrolled nurses and district enrolled nurses**
1992/93	7.6%	7.0%
1993/94	8.8%	8.1%
1994/95	9.2%	10.1%

Note: figures for 1992/93 exclude the S.E. Thames and N.W. Thames RHAs.

Source: Department of Health, KM48 return: joiners and leavers

In April 1996, KM48 was discontinued by the NHS Executive. Official data on nurse turnover and wastage are now collected via two main processes. These are:

- data provided by individual NHS trusts as part of the annual National Balance Sheet exercise (unpublished); and

- data collected by the Office of Manpower Economics (OME) as part of the Nurses and Professionals Allied to Medicine Review Body (NAPRB) Manpower Survey coverage of which was extended to include joiners and leavers data in 1996.

It remains to be seen whether these sources will provide the robust data required for planning purposes. Early indications are not encouraging. Only 52 per cent (n=308) of units made returns on time which were of sufficient quality to be included in the OME's analysis for the Review Body. This compares with a response of 68 per cent in 1995. The OME describe the decline in response as 'disappointing' (Review Body, 1997).

The OME survey showed that 13.7 per cent (21,284) of first and second level registered nursing staff in post had changed jobs in the year to 31 March 1996[8]. Although the survey sought to collect data on the type of leaver (retirement, redundancy, dismissal, transfer *etc.*), more than half (53 per cent) were classed as 'other/don't know'. It would therefore be unwise to distinguish those changing jobs within the NHS and those leaving NHS nursing (wastage).

The OME assert that the wastage rate (leavers *excluding* transfers to other NHS units, as a proportion of staff in post) was 9 per cent for GB, ranging from 14 per cent in North Thames to 5 per cent in Wales. This assumes that none of those whose destination was recorded as 'other/don't know', actually moved to another NHS nursing or nurse management job. These figures are for all nursing staff; the published data do not permit a separate analysis for registered staff only. The total leaving rate (including transfers between NHS units) ranged from 22 per cent in North Thames to 8 per cent in Wales. Turnover was particularly high in Inner London, with one-third of nursing staff changing post or leaving the NHS.

Turnover (*ie* all leavers) was highest among 'other first level nurses'[9] and registered sick children's nurses (whether working in paediatrics or not) at 17.2 per cent and 16.2 per cent respectively, and lowest amongst health visitors and district nurses (both 9 per cent).

The annual IES/RCN surveys provide additional independent, national data on turnover and wastage. However, because of the sample composition (which consists of nurses in RCN membership), it has a tendency to underestimate *wastage* rates. Nevertheless, it has the merits of detail and consistency in definition which other sources lack, and gives robust trend data for the last eight years.

4.3 Turnover and wastage from NHS nursing

Figure 4.1 shows the trend in NHS nurse turnover as recorded by the IES/RCN surveys since the late 1980s.

More than one in five (21 per cent) NHS nurses reported that they had changed jobs or stopped working during 1996-97. The rate of turnover has remained almost unchanged from its 1995-96 level. A total of 22 per cent of respondents who were in NHS nursing posts a year ago, changed jobs or stopped working during 1995-1996. This compares with a figure of 20 per cent during 1994-1995 and 15 per cent during 1993-1994.

Figure 4.1 Turnover among NHS nurses, 1988-89 to 1996-97

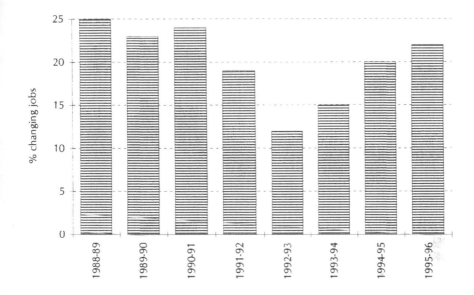

Source: Seccombe and Smith, 1997a

This headline turnover figure includes moves within the NHS as well as moves between the NHS and other employment sectors, and those leaving paid employment altogether. This is a minimum figure, since a proportion (unknown) of those changing jobs and of those leaving nursing may leave RCN membership at the same time and so would be excluded from the sample. Additionally, the sample excluded those who were known to be retired at the time of selection.

Inevitably, most of this turnover is accounted for by nurses moving between different posts within the NHS (see Table 4.2). In each of the surveys, the majority of NHS nurses who changed jobs remained in the NHS. One-third (32 per cent) of the NHS nurses who moved to new posts in the last year also changed employer. The comparable figures for 1995 and 1996 were 27 per cent and 37 per cent respectively. An increase in the proportion of job changes which involves moves between NHS trusts, rather than changes within trusts, suggests that there is a growth in labour market 'churning', particularly since comparatively few of these job moves seem to be accompanied by grade changes.

Table 4.2   Employment status of NHS nurses who changed jobs during 1993-94 to 1996-97

Employment status	1993-94	1994-95	1995-96	1996-97
	%	%	%	%
Moves within the NHS:	**75**	**79**	**78**	**72**
in NHS nursing	n.a.	75	73	68
to NHS management/education	n.a.	4	1	n.a.
to statutory maternity leave	n.a.	-	4	4
Moves from the NHS to:	**25**	**21**	**22**	**28**
Non-NHS nursing	8	7	5	8
Retired	2	2	4	3
Bank nursing	4	3	3	4
Career break	1	1	2	2
Non-nursing jobs	4	2	1	2
Agency nursing	1	1	1	2
Nurse education	-	-	1	2
GP practice nursing	3	2	1	1
Unemployed but seeking work	-	-	>1	>1
Other /imprecise	2	3	2	4

Source: IES/RCN Membership Surveys (various years)

Within this overall picture, there are wide geographical differences which reflect local and regional labour market conditions. Gray *et al (*1988) have shown, for example, that local unemployment levels and the number of registered nursing homes in an area affect turnover amongst nurses. However, such factors are reported to explain only about half the variation in turnover and large differences between nurse employers in the same local labour market remain. This variation must be mainly due to differences in the employment practices of these employers.

The increasing volatility of the nursing labour market may reflect growing demand for registered nurses from a combination of factors including:

•   increased wastage (*eg* due to an increase in retirements or flows to non-NHS employment);

•   a growth in the demand for high quality nursing inputs; and

- shortfalls in supply (returners or newly registered).

The evidence from the IES/RCN surveys and other independent sources suggest that all three factors may be converging.

The 1997 IES/RCN survey also showed a particularly high rate of job change among newly qualified nurses. A third of those who first registered in the last three years changed jobs in the last 12 months.

These data also consistently show that rates of turnover and wastage are higher among younger nurses. In 1996 to 1997 for example, 29 per cent of those aged 25 to 29 changed jobs compared with 9 per cent of those aged 50 to 54 (see Figure 4.2).

Figure 4.2 Proportion of nurses who changed jobs during 1995 to 1996, by age group

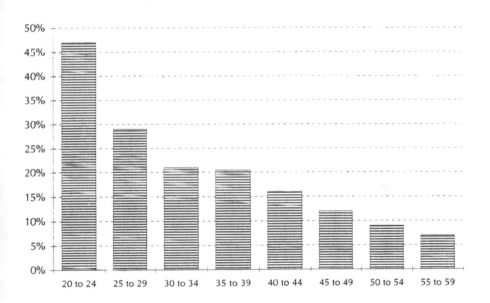

Source: IES/1997 RCN Membership Survey

The reasons why nurses leave their jobs are many and complex. Research (*eg* Irvine and Evans, 1992) consistently shows that most voluntary leavers go because of dissatisfaction with their current employment, rather than because of the attractions of the new job. An increase in the availability of employment makes it more likely that dissatisfied staff will be able to leave.

Table 4.3 shows the reasons stated by NHS nurses for moving between NHS jobs during 1995 to 1996. Positive reasons, including promotion and the desire to develop new skills, account for about 40 per cent of these moves. These proportions are similar to those found in earlier IES/RCN surveys. Such 'career motivators' were also reported to play an important part in decisions by senior managers to move between NHS organisations (Dixon *et al*, 1994). Other, less positive, causes account for nearly a third of moves. These include: job dissatisfaction (16 per cent); ill-health and injury (7 per cent); unit or ward closure (5 per cent); end of temporary contract (2 per cent).

Table 4.3 Main reason for changing jobs within the NHS, during 1995 to 1996

Reason	%
Promotion	25
Dissatisfaction	16
To develop new skills	15
Ill-health/injury	7
Moved from area	5
Further training/additional qualification	5
Unit/ward closure and redundancy	5
Change of working hours	3
End of temporary contract	2
Secondment	1
Other	16

Base number = 362

Source: Seccombe and Smith, 1996

Data from 1997 IES/RCN membership survey confirms this pattern. Dissatisfaction, working hours and stress are cited as the single most important factor in job change by more than two-fifths of respondents.

These survey data also show that wastage from NHS nursing is rising. In 1995 to 1996, just under 6 per cent of those who were in NHS nursing one year ago had left at the time of the survey. This compares with figures of 5 per cent during 1994 to 1995, and 4 per cent during 1993 to 1994 and 1992 to 1993. Again, these should be regarded as minimum figures.

Of those nurses who left NHS nursing during 1995 to 1996, half remained in direct care nursing jobs, including agency and bank nursing (19 per cent), GP practice nursing jobs (6 per cent), independent sector nursing (25 per cent). Table 4.4 shows that during the 1990s the proportion of those leaving the NHS for non-NHS nursing has steadily reduced, while those taking retirement has risen.

Table 4.4   Employment status of those leaving the NHS, 1992-93 to 1995-96

Employment status	1992-93	1993-94	1994-95	1995-96
	%	%	%	%
Non-NHS nursing	34	32	29	25
Bank/agency nursing	17	18	21	19
Retirement	12	8	10	17
Career breaks	13	4	8	10
GP practice nursing	6	10	10	6
Non-nursing work	9	14	9	6
Unemployed	8	5	2	3
Other	2	9	11	14

Source: IES/RCN Membership Surveys (various years)

4.4 Reasons for leaving

The IES/RCN surveys also provide an insight into the reasons why nurses leave the NHS.

The responses of those who left NHS nursing (excluding those on statutory maternity leave) during 1995 to 1996, are given in Table 4.5. Nearly a quarter (23 per cent) of these leavers indicated that job dissatisfaction was their main reason for leaving, with 15 per cent reporting ill health or injury, 10 per cent wanting to develop new skills, and 11 per cent retiring. The reasons for leaving the NHS, cited by nurses, have shown comparatively little variation over the 1990s. Two notable trends have been: an increase (from one in six to one in four)   the proportion giving ill-health, injury or retirement as their reason for leaving; a similar increase in the proportion giving job dissatisfaction as their reason for leaving.

Table 4.5 Reasons for leaving NHS nursing, during 1995 to 1996

Reason	%
Dissatisfaction with job	23
Ill-health/injury	15
Retired	11
To develop new skills	10
Promotion	7
Moved from area	7
Redundant	3
End of temporary contract	2
Gained further qualification	2
Downgraded	1
Other	19

Base number = 127

Source: Seccombe and Smith, 1996

Looking more closely at those who cited 'job dissatisfaction' as their reason for leaving the NHS, we find two significant patterns. Firstly, the majority (71 per cent) are now in nursing jobs outside the NHS. This suggests that it is not nursing itself which these nurses were dissatisfied with but rather the conditions under which they nursed in the NHS. Secondly, more than a third (37 per cent) of these leavers who reported job dissatisfaction as the reason for leaving had first registered since 1990, compared with 17 per cent of all NHS nursing leavers.

4.5 The non-NHS sector

Turnover and wastage from the non-NHS nursing sector are an important component of change in the supply of nurses to the NHS, since a high proportion of NHS leavers go to non-NHS nursing jobs. As we saw above, a quarter of nurses leaving the NHS went to non-NHS nursing jobs (excluding bank, agency and GP practice nursing). Clearly, growth and turnover in this sector have a knock-on effect on the supply of nurses to the NHS. Equally however, non-NHS nursing is a potential source of recruits into NHS nursing.

In 1996 the non-NHS nursing sector experienced a similar level of overall job change to that of the NHS. One in five nurses responding to the IES/RCN survey reported that they had changed jobs, or stopped paid work altogether, during the previous twelve months. Almost half (47 per cent) of this turnover is accounted for by moves between non-NHS employers. This suggests a comparatively lower (9 per cent) level of turnover within the sector than within NHS nursing.

Table 4.6 shows the current employment of those who were in non-NHS nursing one year ago, and who had changed jobs or stopped working.

Table 4.6   Employment status of non-NHS nurses who changed jobs during 1995 to 1996

Employment status	%
Another non-NHS nursing job	47
NHS nursing	21
Bank nursing	8
Agency nursing	2
GP practice nursing	2
Statutory maternity leave	4
Career break	4
Non-nursing employment	4
Nurse education	1
Other	7

Base number =102

Source: Seccombe and Smith, 1996

NHS nursing was the main destination for leavers from non-NHS nursing, accounting for 21 per cent of all job changes (*ie* a little under 5 per cent of those in non-NHS nursing one year ago moved to NHS nursing jobs). Despite this, the NHS was a net loser; the number of nurses moving from NHS to non-NHS nursing employment was more than double the number who moved from non-NHS nursing to NHS nursing employment. The other main destination of those who remained in nursing employment was bank and agency work (10 per cent).

Table 4.7 shows the main reasons given by non-NHS nursing respondents for their job change. Job dissatisfaction was cited by more than two-fifths (41 per cent), followed by moved away from the area (13 per cent) and, to develop new skills (12 per cent).

Table 4.7 Non-NHS nurses: reasons for changing jobs during 1995 to 1996

Reason	%
Job dissatisfaction	41
Moved from area	13
To develop new skills	12
Promotion	11
To change working hours	4
Ill-health or injury	3
Redundancy	3
End of temporary contract	1
Other	12
Base number = 79	

Source: Seccombe and Smith, 1996

Turning finally to those nurses in GP practice employment, we find that turnover was lower than in the other sectors. Only 8 per cent of those who were in GP practice nursing reported changing jobs or stopping work altogether between 1995 and 1996. More than two-fifths of this turnover is accounted for by statutory maternity leave (28 per cent), career breaks (8 per cent), and retirement (8 per cent). Just over a quarter (28 per cent) of job changes involved moves to NHS nursing. There appears to be comparatively little movement of GP practice nurses between practices; less than 4 per cent reported having changed employer within the sector.

4.6 Turnover intentions and morale

One of the key factors in determining the future requirement of nurses in the NHS is the likely level of future wastage from the NHS to other forms of employment. The evidence presented earlier shows that both turnover and wastage are increasing. In this section we present survey evidence on the turnover and leaving intentions of NHS nurses and their perceptions of the desirability of leaving nursing.

Nurses were asked in 1996 to indicate what they thought they would be doing in two years' time. The responses of NHS nurses are shown on Figure 4.3.

Figure 4.3 NHS nurses' anticipated employment in 1998

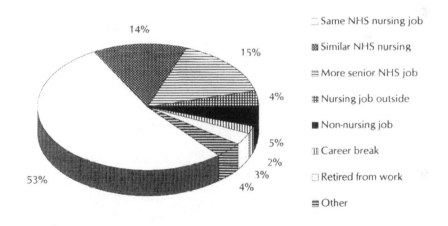

Source: Seccombe and Smith, 1996

Around half (53 per cent) expected to be in the same NHS job with one in seven (14 per cent) saying that they expected to be in a similar job but in a different NHS trust. Only 15 per cent thought that they would be in a more senior NHS job.

Nearly one in five (18 per cent) respondents reported that they expected to leave the NHS within two years. This is similar to the figure reported in the previous year's survey (when 20 per cent reported that they expected to leave) but it is double the 1988 figure. Among those who expect to leave NHS nursing, 4 per cent expected to be in a non-NHS nursing job and 5 per cent in a non-nursing job. Most of the remainder anticipated retirement (3 per cent), taking a career break (2 per cent), entering further education or working abroad.

Turnover intention has frequently been cited as a good indicator of morale in organisations. In particular, low levels of job satisfaction have been shown to influence stated intention to leave. One way of gauging the extent to which nurses perceive leaving the profession as desirable or not, is to examine the extent to which they agree or disagree with the statement '*I would leave nursing if I could*'.

Figure 4.4 compares the responses of NHS nurses to this statement in 1997 with those of the previous four surveys. In 1993, a quarter of NHS respondents agreed or agreed strongly with the statement that '*I would leave nursing if I could*'. This proportion has increased in each of the subsequent surveys, reaching nearly two-fifths (38 per cent) in 1996. The 1997 figure shows a slight downturn from 1996, with 36 per cent agreeing or agreeing strongly. Further, the proportion who agreed strongly has grown from just under 10 per cent in 1993 to 15 per cent in 1995 and 17 per cent in 1996.

Figure 4.4 'I would leave nursing if I could': NHS nurses, 1993 to 1997

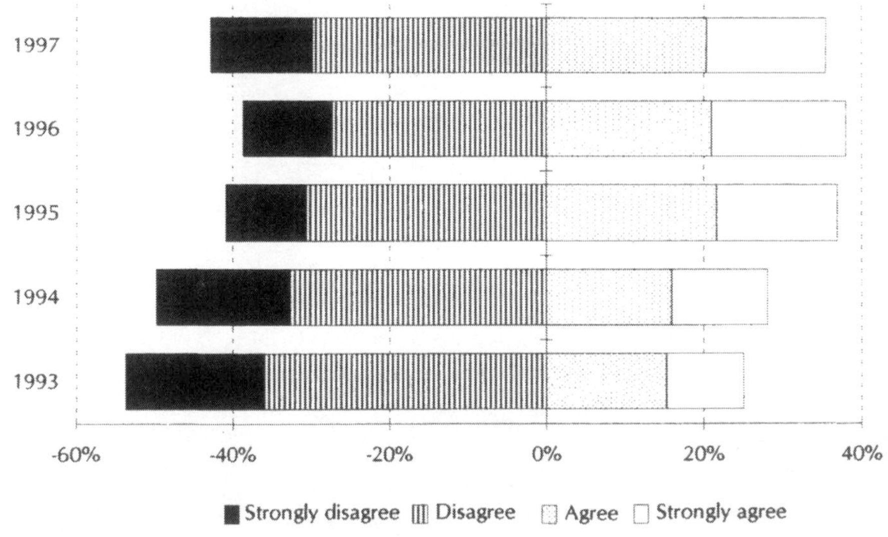

Source: Seccombe and Smith, 1997a

Further analysis shows that turnover intention, using this measure, is higher among acute hospital based nurses (40 per cent), than among those in non-acute hospital (35 per cent) or community settings (32 per cent).

Figure 4.5 shows that NHS nurses were more likely to agree with the statement than GP practice nurses and nurses in most other non-NHS nursing employment. Agency nurses were, however, the group most likely to agree with the statement.

Figure 4.5 Proportion of nurses who agreed 'I would leave nursing if I could', by employment sector

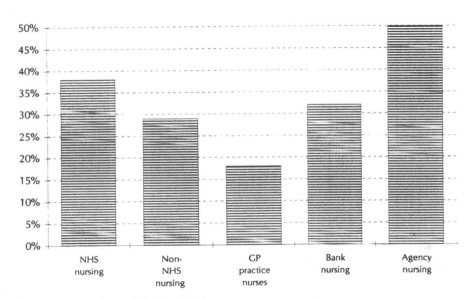

Source: Seccombe and Smith, 1996

Overall, these data suggest that for a high proportion of nurses, particularly those in NHS nursing, there is a significant mismatch between the rewards (including management style, career prospects, working hours) offered by the work environment, and their needs and expectations. As a result, they tend to agree that they would leave nursing if they could. However, the extent to which they are able to do so is determined by external job opportunities and their own personal and domestic circumstances. Thus 38 per cent of NHS nurses agreed with the statement that '*I would leave nursing if I could*' but only 13 per cent actually expect to be in non-nursing employment or not in employment altogether, in two years' time.

4.7 Summary

The NHS faces a short to medium-term fall in the availability of newly qualified nurses, with increasing opportunities for non-NHS employment, and an already high participation rates in nursing employment. Identifying and implementing effective retention policies has again assumed a more prominent position on trust management agendas.

The key findings presented in this chapter include:

- turnover in NHS nursing has increased since the early 1990s and appears to have stabilised; 21 per cent of NHS nurses changed jobs or stopped working in 1996/97;

- the NHS nursing labour market is becoming more volatile — 32 per cent of those NHS nurses who changed jobs in 1996-97 also changed employers;

- job dissatisfaction, ill-health and injury have become increasingly prevalent as reasons for job change;

- wastage from NHS nursing has also increased;

- retirement, early retirement and ill-health retirement account for an increasing proportion of leavers;

- in 1996, one in five NHS nurses expected to leave the service by 1998; few anticipated career progression within the NHS;

- both turnover and wastage are comparatively lower in non-NHS nursing, and lowest among GP practice nurses; and

- the NHS 'loses' two nurses to non-NHS nursing employment, for each one it recruits back.

5 Nurses' Pay

5.1 Introduction

This chapter examines nurses' pay in relation to the dynamics of the UK nursing labour market. It focuses particularly on the situation since the establishment of the Review Body in 1983, and the debate on the potential use of local pay determination for NHS nurses.

Despite its perceived importance as a mechanism for recruiting, retaining and motivating staff, the precise role of pay in influencing employee behaviour has rarely been examined in isolation from other factors, either in nursing or any other occupation. There is no generally accepted model of the relationship between pay and recruitment, turnover or performance, and little empirical evidence to assist in determining such a model.

As noted elsewhere in this book, much of the recurring concern about shortages of nursing staff, in Britain and elsewhere, has focused on pay - either low pay as a causal factor, or improved pay as a solution. Several of the major 'official' scrutinies of UK nursing (eg Halsbury, 1974) have arisen as a result of concerns about the relative and absolute level of nurses' pay. It has been argued in several of these reports that comparatively low pay rates in nursing have acted as a disincentive to enter the profession, have caused high turnover rates, and are related to low morale and de-motivation of staff. This argument is evident in reports dating back to the 1930s (Lancet, 1932).

Whilst the argument linking 'low' pay rates to nurses' morale and motivation is superficially persuasive, it has to be viewed within the context of the labour market characteristics and behaviour of nurses. The monopsony effect that the NHS may have had on pay levels also has to be considered. The aim of this chapter is to review relevant published research, report on survey results that have examined UK nurses' attitudes to pay, and examine the likely labour market effects of changes in the way that NHS nurses' pay is determined.

5.2 Trends in pay determination in UK nursing

Until recently, NHS nurses' pay had always been determined at a national level. From the creation of the NHS in 1948, until the establishment of the Review Body in 1983, the determination of nurses' pay was the responsibility of the Nurses and Midwives Whitley Council. Representatives of the Staff (the unions and professional organisations) and Management Sides (the Departments of Health and NHS management) met regularly to negotiate pay structures and pay increases as well as to agree other terms and conditions of employment.

The inability of the Whitley Council to reach agreement often led to arbitration or to the involvement of the Industrial Court in the 1950s and 1960s (the court made eight awards related to nurses' pay between December 1952 and 1956) (Gray, 1989). The absence of well-defined separate governmental and NHS management roles in the Whitley machinery, and the lack of direct involvement (but indirect influence) of the Treasury, were contributory factors to these recurring difficulties. Low pay increases were the end result for a number of years, and there was frequent recourse to special reviews to relieve the tension in the system and to allow nurses' pay levels to be improved. There were four such 'special reviews' in the 1960s (Halsbury, 1974).

These 'catching up' exercises were symptomatic of the difficulties of resolving tensions within the Whitley system, and, as the term 'special review' suggests, were primarily intended to secure reinstatement of a previous level of 'real pay', rather than any actual improvements in pay, in comparison with other occupations.

The first independent (*ie* non-Whitley) review of NHS nurses' pay was conducted in 1967-68, by the National Board of Prices and Incomes (NBPI). The NBPI review was followed by other independent reviews in 1974 (Halsbury) and 1979-80 (Clegg). Table 5.1 shows the key features of each review. Each review was a one-off exercise, which had an immediate positive effect on levels of pay. The effects of the reviews were then eroded in the following few years.

This 'stop-go' situation was finally ended in 1983, with the establishment of a Review Body, to 'advise the Prime Minister' on the pay of Nurses, Midwives and Health Visitors (including unqualified nursing auxiliaries, and nurse learners). The government made the commitment that '*successive governments have agreed to accept Review Body recommendations unless there are clear and compelling reasons for not*

Table 5.1 National review of nurses' pay, 1968 to 1988

1968	National Board for Prices and Incomes	First independent inquiry into nurses' pay since 1948. The Board had to observe government pay restraint measures. Broad ranging recommendations included improving 'efficiency' by better deployment of staff and revised shift patterns. Pay increases aimed at raising differentials and to combat shortages in specific areas, particularly at staff nurse level.
1970	Whitley Council (Internal Review)	Special review which recommended substantial increases in pay - primarily as a catching up exercise. Minor alterations to pay structure.
1974	Committee of Inquiry (Halsbury)	Second independent inquiry. It concluded that nurses pay had 'fallen behind' other occupations since 1970. It proposed significant increases in pay to 'catch up' and to combat staff shortages. It also proposed 'simplifying' the pay/grading structures.
1980	Standing Commission on Pay Comparability (Clegg)	Third major independent review on nurses' pay. Recommendations were based on factor analysis of job evaluation. It recommended a reduction in working hours to 37.5 hours per week. It recommended a major pay uplift as pay levels had fallen since Halsbury. Also voiced concern about danger of future erosion of its recommendations.
1983 to Current	Review Body	Annual recommendations on pay levels, from 1984 onwards. It receives evidence from the Management and Staff Sides of Whitley Council. The government is committed to implementing recommendations, unless there are 'clear and compelling' reasons otherwise. Traditionally, the Review Body has dealt only with pay, but in recent years it has attempted to broaden its remit.
1987-88	Clinical Grading Review - Whitley Council (Internal Review)	A new pay/grading structure for clinical grades was established based on job analysis. This structure was then 'priced' by the Review Body.

Source: Buchan, 1992

doing so'. The Review Body, in its first Report (1984), stressed its 'major advantage' over previous committees:

> 'We are a standing body, and will be keeping the pay of nursing staff under review continuously from year to year. We shall therefore be able progressively to take account of a wide range of factors including job content and organisation, pay developments elsewhere, and changing economic circumstances.'

It has followed an annual cycle of work, receiving and reviewing evidence late in one calendar year, and forwarding its recommendations to government and publishing its report in the following year, with an implementation date of 1 April. The main issues which it has indicated it will consider are:

- 'affordability' — economic and financial considerations;

- recruitment and retention including vacancy rates, turnover rates and the supply of and demand for staff;

- 'fairness' and comparability — pay and earnings data in the NHS and elsewhere are reviewed;

- morale and motivation — general consideration is given to issues related to job satisfaction; and

- productivity and workload — indicators of 'productivity' and changes in workload of staff are reviewed.

The Review Body (1990) stated that it would continue to take account of any further information which became available up to the month of December preceding its recommendations in February/March. It acknowledged that this would lead to fluctuations, which would 'even themselves out' from year to year. Although the government is committed to implementing the Review Body recommendations, in practice, it has often 'staged' or delayed 'full' pay rises in order to reduce total costs.

Arguably there may be a 'simpler' method for determining nurses' pay, other than that of the Review Body. The indexation of police and firefighter pay, using formulae index-linked to increases in earnings, can be cited as working examples of public sector pay determination without recourse to independent bodies. The Review Body is, however, independent and its response can be flexible. It is not an automatic mechanism. It may decide, for instance, to recommend increases in any one year that are at variance with the 'going rate' determined by a mechanistic formula.

Between 1983 and 1995, the Review Body recommendations were based on pay uplifts and alterations of pay differentials at national level. Meanwhile the management side argued for a move to local pay determination. In 1995, the Review Body recommended that a significant element of local control and flexibility be introduced in the allocating the nursing paybill.

The role of the Review Body as custodian of a national pay and grading structure was significantly eroded by these recommendations in 1995, which signalled the first move towards a major element of local pay determination for NHS nurses. The subsequent recommendations of the 1996 report changed the focus of pay determination from a national to a local level. A greater emphasis was placed on the 'X plus Y' approach (X=national, Y=local), and for local agreement on the 'Y' element of the local pay award. If these 'X plus Y' awards had continued in subsequent years, the central role of the Review Body would have reduced as local management took on increasing responsibility for allocating the 'Y' element of the paybill.

However, in 1997 the Review Body recommended a national award after criticising the capability of many trusts to deliver local pay. It also restated its commitment, in principal, to using some element of local pay.

Figure 5.1 illustrates the trend in the average gross weekly earnings of nurses in full-time employment as a percentage of average non-manual earnings, between 1984 and 1997. In the mid to late 1980s nurses' earnings were comparatively stable, fluctuating between 72 and 74 per cent of average non-manual earnings. Following the clinical grading review in 1988, there was an increase in nurses' relative earnings to 84 per cent of the non-manual average. In the first half of the 1990s the relative earnings of nurses continued to exhibit small year-on-year fluctuations, but showed no real improvement over the 1989 figure.

Examination of longer term trends in nurses' earnings showed fluctuations in comparative earnings levels in the 1970s and early 1980s and a period of comparative stability in the second half of the 1980s and early 1990s. Elliot and Duffus (1996), showed that in 1992, registered nurses were lying 19th (male) and 22nd (female) in a ranking of 44 public service sector occupations.

The pay/grading structure for NHS nurses remained basically unaltered for 40 years, from the establishment of the NHS in 1948 until 1988. In that year, a new clinical grading structure was implemented, with new grades being 'priced' by the Review Body. The grading structure and the criteria used to determine grading were developed and agreed by the Nurses and

Figure 5.1   Nurses' earnings during 1984 to 1997 as a proportion of all non-manual earnings

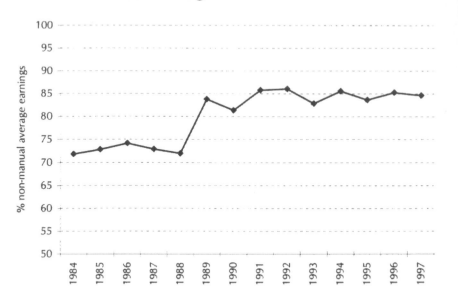

Source: Seccombe and Smith, 1996 (figures updated to include data from 1996 and 1997)

Midwives Whitley Council. Initial work by external management consultants was unacceptable to both sides, and the work was undertaken 'in-house', using management and staff nominees to conduct fieldwork interviews of several hundred nurses, and to reach agreement on the criteria and structure.

The implementation of clinical grading was not without problems (see Beardshaw and Robinson, 1990). Many were linked to the excessively 'positive' marketing of the scheme and the potential difficulties of determining the costs of funding clinical grading prior to its implementation (Buchan, 1988). The application of differential pay increases to individual nurses at a local level caused discontent. Differences in interpretation of this criteria, or in the application of clinical grading, created varying patterns of clinical grading in different employing units. As a consequence many NHS nurses appealed against their grade outcome. The appeals procedure could not cope with the large number of appellants. It took many years for some nurses to secure a hearing.

In its 1992 report, the Review Body noted:

'Over 30,000 appeals arising from the 1988 clinical grading review are still waiting to be heard. Dissatisfaction about the backlog has infected the attitude of many staff to the pay scales themselves' (para 12).

The Review Body was critical of parts of the process of management involvement in the initial grading process (1989, para 5). Survey data showed that, in 1988, approximately 30 per cent of qualified nurses were very dissatisfied with the outcome of clinical grading. A 'follow up' survey showed an overall improvement in satisfaction (see Figure 5.2).

Figure 5.2 Satisfaction with clinical grading amongst qualified nurses, 1988 and 1990

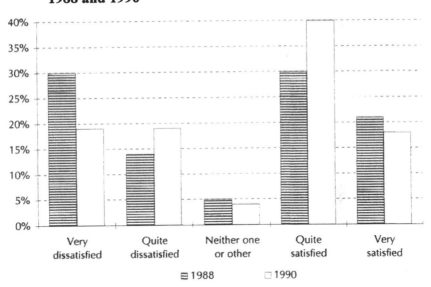

Source: Buchan, 1992

Since the implementation of clinical grading in 1988 there have been other developments in relation to NHS nurses' pay. These are: Department of Health led attempts to pilot local pay supplements in the late 1980s (see section 5.2.1); the use of performance related pay (PRP) in nursing in the early 1990s (see section 5.2.2); and the gradual attempt to introduce local pay in the mid-1990s (see section 5.2.3).

5.2.1 Local pay supplements

As noted in the introductory chapter, one of the key outcomes of the NHS reforms was to increase the autonomy of employing units. NHS trusts were to have the opportunity to determine pay locally, rather than rely on central national negotiations. An early attempt to encourage the use of local pay was undertaken by the Department of Health (England) in 1988/89. The Department made available a comparatively small amount of funding (£5 million in the first year) to provide pay supplements of up to £1,000 per annum for 'hard to fill' posts. Analysis of the first year of the scheme, which covered 7,164 posts (Buchan, 1989), found that the regional distribution of bids for the pay supplements was geographically skewed; some regions with reported recruitment difficulties did not participate in the exercise.

Subsequently, the Department of Health requested that the Review Body extend the scheme, but the Review Body declined, stating that it required further evidence of the cost effectiveness of the scheme. In its 1991 report, the Review Body was critical of evaluation of the scheme, and concluded that no firm conclusions on its impact could be drawn. The scheme was then subsumed within general discussions between management and staff sides on the introduction of local pay.

5.2.2 Performance related pay

Performance related pay (PRP) for individual employees was in vogue in the early 1990s, as a mechanism for improving 'productivity' in the public sector, under the Conservative government of the time. The emphasis on improving quality in public services was highlighted in the government's Citizen's Charter, which made explicit reference to the introduction of a greater element of PRP as a method of securing value for money for the taxpayer, whilst retaining tight cost control. In practice, the extension of the use of individual PRP to clinically based staff in the NHS was extremely limited, with only a handful of NHS trusts making any real attempt to link the pay of individual nurses directly to any 'measure' of 'performance'.

The potential for using PRP in UK nursing labour markets was reviewed by Thompson and Buchan (1993). Drawing on evidence from other sectors and from nursing in the US, they concluded that any attempt to implement the traditional form of appraisal-based individual PRP for nurses in the NHS would be highly problematic. They cited the administrative workload of reviewing individual performance for pay determination purposes, the difficulties of objectively 'measuring' individual nurses' work and performance as most worked in multi-disciplinary teams, and the lack of evidence of long term sustainability of the link between individual PRP and organisational performance as constraining factors. Individual performance related pay has not, in practice, become a factor of any significance for most NHS nurses, although at one time it was high on the governments agenda. Trends and managerial focus on pay determination have moved on towards skills and competence based pay (see, *for example,* NHS Personnel, 1996; Buchan and Thompson, 1997).

5.2.3 *'Real' local pay*

The NHS reform-led introduction of locally based pay determination for NHS nurses was characterised by the slow, and often uncertain pace of implementation. Major constraints on the implementation of local pay included the following: the initial absence of local bargaining structures and local level management skills in pay determination; funding limitations; and a lack of political (and in some cases managerial) will to push for rapid change (see Buchan, 1992; Buchan and Seccombe, 1994; Bach and Winchester, 1994). After a number of years of 'phoney war', with little real activity in local pay determination for the majority of NHS nurses, the pace of change increased when the Review Body published its 1995 report.

This 1995 report signalled the introduction of a local element of pay determination for all NHS nurses. The first year of the application of this approach did not lead to much variation between trusts in pay settlements. However, it did mark the beginning of 'real' activity on pay determination at local level, and provided a stimulus for all NHS trusts to make at least a cursory attempt at examining how to introduce an element of pay at a local level. In 1996 the Review Body gave further impetus to local pay, by weighting the overall pay award heavily in favour of the 'Y' local element (in contrast to very different treatment for doctors, where pay determination has been retained at national level).

However, the limited funding available for the local pay element gave little room for manoeuvre for local managers (even those keen on taking the initiative on local pay) and restricted the extent of variation of pay settlements between NHS trusts. Management side evidence to the Review Body in 1997 marked a *volte-face* in their perspective on local pay. In previous years they had argued that local pay was important in solving local recruitment difficulties. In 1996/97 they adopted a different position, arguing that local pay should *not* be used to address shortages, as this could lead to a pay spiral.

Whilst there was increased activity at local level on pay determination in the years 1995-97, there was little action, in terms of developing new pay structures or approaches to nurses' pay determination. Few NHS trusts tried, and fewer succeeded, in replacing the standard 'Whitley' template as a means of paying the majority of their nursing staff. The few exceptions include a small number of trusts which introduced a 'single pay spine', linked to job evaluation for all staff *(eg* South Tees NHS Trust), or introduced appraisal based payment systems (Derby NHS Trust), or piloted competency based pay/grading (Ealing NHS Trust).

However, for every NHS trust which rose to prominence because it was trying out a novel or radical approach, there were many others where resources or willpower were not sufficient to drive through the radical change envisaged by the architects of the NHS reforms. Most NHS nurses remain on Whitley terms and conditions of employment. The Review Body noted in its 1997 Report that at trust level, resources and will-power had often been lacking, and recommended a national award, with no local element. The election of a new Labour government in May 1997 would appear to have stopped the move towards completely devolved pay determination.

Key issues to be resolved under the new government included: the retention of separate Review Bodies or pay 'spines' for different health professional groups; the need to sustain equal pay for equal work; and the implications of any minimum wage legislation on the pay of NHS nurses.

The future for nurses' pay in the NHS appears to be linked to broader decisions from government on what should constitute 'flexibility in pay determination and employment practice'. It may be that this 'flexibility' will be pursued by managers at local level focusing more on achieving cost savings through changes in working patterns and associated conditions of employment, than through a direct attempt at introducing local (non 'Whitley') pay rates (see *eg* Buchan, 1994a). Another possibility is that a combination of national and local pay determination, associated with an actual or notional 'minimum wage', will lead to a narrowing of pay differentials between qualified nurses and nursing auxiliaries. This would reverse the trend set by the Review Body which increased differentials in the late 1980s.

The extent to which pay levels and any local pay variation may impact on the labour market behaviour of nurses is examined below.

5.3 Research on pay and nurses' labour market behaviour

This section reviews the limited research on pay and nurses' labour market behaviour, the effects of unionisation and monopsony on nurses' pay, and the links between nurses' pay and job satisfaction.

5.3.1 Pay and labour market behaviour

Research on the relationship between pay and labour market characteristics of nurses in Britain can only be regarded as exploratory, with few examples existing on which to make any firm conclusions. Hoskins (1982) used regression analysis to establish tentative links between the supply of nursing and midwifery staff and pay rates. He claimed that '*the rate at which midwives leave their work, and hence the total stock of midwives, is sensitive to pay changes*'.

Gray *et al* (1988) researched the links between nurse turnover and a number of local labour market variables *(eg* unemployment rates). Using regression analysis, they identified how much of the variation in nurse turnover could be explained by local labour market conditions. The definition of local labour markets used in the study was the standard 'travel to work' area. They claimed to find a significant relationship between turnover rates and three variables - local unemployment, size of the private nursing home sector, and level of non-manual female earnings. The study did not explain all of the variation between staff turnover of different groups and labour markets. It did point to the influence of local labour market factors on nurses' behaviour in the labour market (see also Gray and Phillips, 1996).

In an overview of the NHS and the labour market, Wilson and Stilwell (1992) considered the impact of pay rates on labour market behaviour. On the basis of the limited research available, they concluded that:

'What seems beyond doubt is that economic factors do influence nursing supply' (p.121).

They argued that the few available studies (most from the US) gave indications of '*strong positive wage elasticity*' and that:

'increases in NHS pay levels will significantly help overcome shortages of female labour by attracting new recruits of all ages, by reducing the quit rate of existing employees, and by accelerating the return of currently inactive past employees' (p.92).

They also highlighted the need for further UK research in this area.

The relationship between nurses' pay and labour market characteristics has been researched more in the United States than in Britain. For example, research has been conducted on the following topics: the effect of unionisation on nurses' pay; the links between monopsony power and pay levels; and the relationship between pay rates and participation rates in employment.

In terms of the age profile, participation in employment, a high prevalence of part-time working, and a high proportion of female nurses, the characteristics of the US nursing workforce are similar to those in the UK (Buchan, 1992). The US, however, differs from Britain with regard to two aspects of nurses' pay determination. First, there has never been co-ordinated national pay determination in the US. Nurses' pay has normally been set at hospital level. Secondly, the unionisation of nurses has been lower in the US, and it has varied markedly between different hospitals, states and regions.

5.3.2 The 'union' effect

The majority of nurses in the United States work in non-unionised workplaces. Some US researchers have found evidence that suggests a link between the existence of union representation and collective bargaining and higher pay rates for nurses. Becker, Sloan and Steinwald (1982) conducted a large study which suggested that the 'union' effect increased wages by 6 per cent for registered nurses (RNs) in comparison with non-unionised nurses. The same study found evidence of higher pay increases in hospitals where work stoppages had occurred. Brider (1991) reported that the 'union effect' adds five to 7 per cent to the salary of qualified nurses.

5.3.3 Monopsony

Some studies from the US have lent support to the theory that there is a monopsony effect at work in many nursing labour markets. It has been argued that in a labour market where there is only one significant employer of nurses (monopsony), or where there is a small number of employers (oligopsony), the comparative lack of competition limits the effect of market adjustments on pay levels. The 'free market' may exist, but there is only one buyer of labour who can set the 'going rate', or a small group of buyers, who may collude to maintain pay levels at a level below that which would be dictated by the 'market'.

One aspect of nurses' pay determination in the United States which has particular relevance to the NHS is the organisational and labour market impact of local pay. Miller, Becker and Krinsky (1979), found that where multiple bargaining units existed (*ie* where employers formed an association to maintain pay levels), lower salary costs ensued more commonly than in single bargaining units:

> 'This bargaining structure tends to reduce much of the internal whipsawing that might prevail in single employer bargaining, and apparently provides sufficient countervailing power to minimise union gains' (p.101).

The same argument, from a different perspective, was promoted by Cleland (1990). She argued that unionisation of nurses acted as a countervailing force to monopsony-based employer wage-setting cartels.

The effect of monopsony in suppressing nurse pay rates in the United States was cited as a major factor in creating the nursing shortages evident in the 1960s and 1970s. One researcher (Yett, 1970) conducted a survey of the 31 largest hospital associations in the United States to determine whether or not they ran 'wage stabilisation' programmes. Fourteen of the fifteen hospital associations which responded to his survey indicated that they did co-operate in some form of wage setting, whilst the fifteenth asked for advice on how to establish a wage stabilisation programme. More recent examples of employer collusion to maintain nurse pay rates in the United States have been reported by Friss (1987) and Cleland (1990), and other researchers (*eg* Link and Landon, 1975; Booton and Lane, 1985) have claimed to find evidence of a monopsony effect on nurse pay levels. It should be noted that there is no overall consistency in the findings of US research in this area. Other studies (*eg* Hirsch and Schumacher, 1995) report little evidence of monopsony in US nursing labour markets.

In recent years, concern about the 'price-fixing' effect of such cartels has led the US Federal government to place restrictions on the conduct and coverage of health sector salary surveys to reduce the 'dampening' effect this can have on pay rates for nurses. In the UK, surveys provided by NHS pay 'clubs' and by management consultants could have a similar constraining effect on any pay variations between NHS trusts.

5.3.4 Participation rates and pay

Buerhaus (1991) examined the wage elasticity of supply of registered nurses in the US (the wage elasticity of supply refers to the extent to which there is a change in labour supply resulting from a change in wage level).

Buerhaus used 1984 data on gender, age, race, marital status, number of children, educational qualifications, hours worked and earnings relating to over 30,000 nurses. He found wage elasticity of 0.49 for married nurses (for every 1 per cent increase in wages, nurses would work an increase of 0.49 per cent in hours worked). The wage elasticity for unmarried RNs was 0.89 - an increase in hours of 0.89 per cent for every additional 1 per cent in pay. In practice Buerhaus suggests that this means 168 more hours per year would be worked by this group in response to an hourly wage increase of $1. The author concluded that:

> 'raising RN wages can be expected to help dynamic shortages by stimulating short run increases in the number of hours worked by currently employed RNs. Moreover, using a wage policy to help bring about a balance between the supply and demand for RNs will help increase the long run supply of RNs by stimulating future enrolment in nursing education programs'.

Similar arguments that increased pay would lead to increased participation in employment had been made by Wilson and Stilwell (1992), and by Phillips (1995) in relation to female nurses in the NHS.

5.3.5 Satisfaction with pay

The above research has adopted primarily a labour economics approach to assessing the impact of nurses' pay. The other discipline and area of research activity which has given some consideration to the links between pay and nurses' labour market behaviour is that drawing from occupational psychology. Most of these studies examine the determinants of job satisfaction and/or 'withdrawal behaviour' from work. They tend to focus on testing behavioural models, are often based on comparatively small and localised data-sets, and have often been inconclusive. Two recently published meta-analyses of research in this area (Blegen, 1993; Irvine and Evans, 1995) provide a useful overview of the current state of knowledge - most of which is based on North American studies.

Blegen (1993) identified over 250 studies examining aspects of nurse job satisfaction, and subjected 42 to meta-analysis. The studies examined in the meta-analysis covered approximately 15,000 nurses in total. The main findings were of a significant negative link between job satisfaction and stress, and a significant positive link between job satisfaction and individual commitment. Other links were with autonomy, communication with supervisors and peers, and (of less significance) fairness in reward distribution. No other link between job satisfaction and pay was identified, because pay was reportedly rarely a factor examined in the studies in the meta-analysis. Blegen suggests that the reason for infrequent examination of the effect of pay was because pay varied so little in the subject groups under examination - these were usually registered nurses in a single work environment, and therefore subject to the same pay determination mechanism.

The more recent meta-analysis by Irvine and Evans (1995), examined causal relationships between job satisfaction, behavioural intentions, and nurse turnover behaviour. They conducted a time series study, covering the period up to 1993, with a cut-off of 1987. The aim was to compare pre- and post-1987 studies to identify whether the effects of a period of nursing shortages (1987-93) were different from those of a 'looser' labour market. Contrary to expectations, the authors found no significant differences between the two time series. The statistically significant results reported by Irvine and Evans were similar to those reported by Blegen; they found the most significant relationships were between job satisfaction and stress, communication with supervisor, autonomy, age and work experience. Pay was not examined by many of the studies reported in the meta-analysis.

In relation to the role of pay on nurses' labour market behaviour, the main conclusions which can be drawn from the two meta-analyses are that factors other than pay clearly can impact on job satisfaction and turnover, and that the effect of pay has not been examined to the extent that allows detailed consideration. What is of some relevance, drawn from Blegen, is that some studies have found evidence of a relationship between job satisfaction of nurses and fairness in reward distribution, which highlights the effect of equity and notions of 'felt-fairness' on individual nurse employees and therefore on reward strategy. It is also significant that the studies, mainly drawn from North America, reportedly have often not examined pay because of a lack of pay variation reported by the samples of nurses examined within employing units.

5.3.6 Lessons from the research

Pay levels in nursing are often regarded as the main reason for labour market problems (because pay is 'low') or are promoted as the main solution to labour market problems (because pay can be increased). The assumption that there is a direct linear relationship between pay rates and labour market behaviour, and therefore that adjusting pay will have a predictable effect on labour market behaviour of nurses, clearly oversimplifies a much more complex issue. The limited research evidence from UK and North America suggests that pay is one of a number of factors which may play a role in shaping or dictating labour market behaviour.

Some of the research reviewed has tentatively confirmed links between pay rates and other factors, such as participation rates and turnover, but the relationship, if positive, has often been found to be weak. In this respect, it has to be acknowledged that nursing does not differ from most other occupational labour markets - there is no commonly accepted and proven model of the role and impact of pay on labour market behaviour.

What can also be taken from the research reviewed above is that the potential for a monopsony effect, the limited geographical mobility of many nurses, and the requirement made of many nurses to achieve a balance between career and domestic commitments ensure that the relationship between nurses' pay and labour market behaviour is a complex one. Some of the relevant research from the US, where pay determination is localised, suggests that employers of nurses often pay below the level which would be dictated by market forces. They can do this because most competition for nurses is often limited to a few major employers, and collusion exists between these employers, through cartels or the informal exchange of information, to maintain pay levels. The establishment of various regional and national pay information 'clubs' and units in the NHS could serve as the forum for information exchange and dampening down of pay variations between NHS trusts. Other US studies indicate that this monopsony effect may be less evident where nurses are unionised and bargain collectively.

5.4 Nurses' pay perceptions

The series of IES/RCN membership surveys enables an examination of trends in pay satisfaction. Over the years respondents have been asked to indicate the extent to which they agree or disagree with a number of attitudinal items concerning relative pay. These items include:

- *I could be paid more for less effort if I left nursing.*

- *Considering the work I do I am paid well.*

- *NHS nurses are paid poorly in relation to other professional groups.*

The first two items have been used in each of the last six surveys. Figure 5.3 summarises the responses of the NHS nurses in the 1997 survey.

Figure 5.3 Summary of pay satisfaction items: NHS nurses, 1997

I could be paid more for less effort if I left nursing	
Considering the work I do I am paid well	
NHS nurses are paid poorly in relation to other professional groups	

-80% -60% -40% -20% 0% 20% 40% 60% 80% 100%

■ Strongly disagree ⦙⦙⦙ Disagree ☐ Agree ☐ Strongly agree

Source: Seccombe and Smith, 1997a

Three-fifths (62 per cent) of NHS nurses surveyed agreed with the statement '*I could be paid more for less effort if I left nursing*'. The proportion agreeing with this statement has increased with each successive survey, having risen from 45 per cent in 1992. Further analysis shows that while similar proportions of male and female nurses agreed with the statement (61 per cent and 62 per cent respectively), over one–third (35 per cent) of male nurses agreed strongly with the statement compared with 30 per cent of female nurses.

Despite this difference by sex (and the disproportionate representation of men in the higher clinical grades), the proportion of NHS nurses who agreed with the statement is inversely related to their clinical grade (see Table 5.2). For example, 63 per cent of D and 65 per cent of E grade nurses agreed or strongly agreed with the statement compared with 58 per cent of G grades and 54 per cent of H grades.

NHS nurses' perception that their relative earnings had declined is shared by most nurses outside the NHS. 61 per cent of non-NHS nurses and 51 per cent of GP practice nurses agreed with the statement.

In relation to the second statement, '*considering the work I do I am paid well*', two-thirds (66 per cent) of NHS nurses rejected this view. This compares with little over half (56 per cent) of those in non-NHS nursing. In contrast, only two-fifths (42 per cent) of GP practice nurses and under half (46 per cent) of those in nurse education disagreed with the statement.

Table 5.2 'Considering the work I do I am paid well': NHS nurses by clinical grade, 1997

	% who				
Grade	Strongly Agree	Agree	Disagree	Strongly Disagree	Base No
D	1	6	43	34	536
E	<1	7	44	29	977
F	1	10	45	25	405
G	2	15	38	19	506
H	1	20	30	14	167

Source: IES/RCN 1997 Membership Survey

Figure 5.4 shows the trend in response for NHS nurses responding over the last six years. In 1997, only 12 per cent of NHS nurses agreed with the

Figure 5.4   'Considering the work I do, I am paid well': NHS nurses, 1992 to 1997

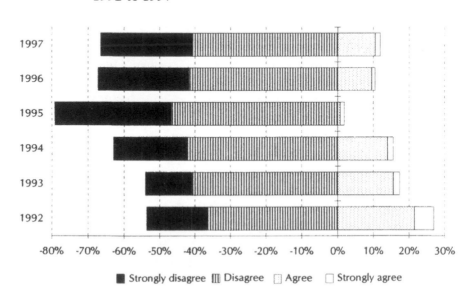

Source: Seccombe and Smith, 1997a

statement, *'considering the work I do I am paid well'*. This is marginally higher than the value for 1996 (10 per cent) but still suggests a substantial deterioration in pay satisfaction during the 1990s. In 1992, for example, 24 per cent of NHS nurses agreed with the statement.

The third statement *'NHS nurses are paid poorly in relation to other professional groups'* was introduced to the survey for the first time in 1995. At that time, 83 per cent agreed, with the statement (58 per cent agreeing strongly). By 1997, the proportion of NHS nurses agreeing with this statement had risen marginally to 85 per cent.

In its Thirteenth report, the Review Body for Nursing Staff commented that:

'It has become clear to us . . . that in general little or no attempt has been made to communicate the benefits of local pay determination to nursing staff, who tend to regard it largely as a cost-cutting exercise. This seems likely to have exacerbated staff fears about the inspiration for, and likely consequences of, local pay' (para 27).

They also noted:

'We believe that Trusts should set out to allay the fears of staff that local pay will lead to lower levels of pay and conditions. The perception that staff could only lose out through local pay determination was a striking feature of our visits' (para 28).

Results of the surveys in 1995 and 1996 suggest that NHS management were unable to alter these perceptions. Respondents to the 1995 RCN membership survey were asked to indicate the extent to which they agreed or disagreed with the following statements about local pay determination:

- *local pay will increase uncertainty about future pay;*
- *local pay bargaining is an appropriate approach to NHS nurses pay;*
- *all nurses should receive the same pay rise;*
- *local pay will mean that high quality nursing is more likely to be rewarded;*
- *local pay will result in unfair deals for some nurses.*

At the time of the 1995 survey, many nurses had not been affected by the process of local pay negotiation or its outcome. One year later, against a backdrop of increased activity on local pay, respondents to the 1996 RCN membership survey were asked once again to indicate the extent of agreement with the same statements on local pay. The overall responses for NHS nurses are summarised in Figure 5.5.

Figure 5.5 Summary of local pay items: NHS nurses, 1996

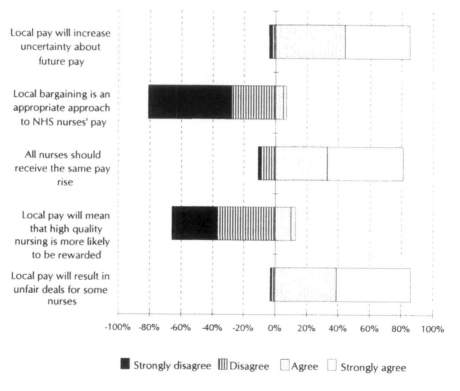

Source: Seccombe and Smith, 1996

In 1996 (as in 1995), the overwhelming majority (85 per cent) of NHS nurses agreed with the statement that *local pay will increase uncertainty about future pay*. The proportion of nurses who disagreed with this statement halved from 8 to 4 per cent. Local bargaining was rejected by most of these nurses as '*an appropriate approach to NHS nurses' pay*'; as in 1995, only 7 per cent of NHS nurses agreed with this statement. Nurses were generally unchanged in their view that local pay will not '*reward high quality nursing*', only 13 per cent agreed with this view.

The majority of respondents agreed that *all nurses should receive the same pay rise*; in fact this proportion increased marginally, from 79 per cent in 1995 to 81 per cent in 1996. Similarly, 86 per cent agreed that '*local pay will result in unfair deals for some nurses*'.

These results indicate that the overwhelming majority of nurses remained unconvinced by the arguments put forward in favour of local pay determination. In 1995, they showed a pronounced lack of enthusiasm for the principle of local pay; in 1996, they also rejected it from experience. The results of the 1996 survey suggested that managers had failed to allay the fears alluded to by the Review Body, and also highlighted the extent to which individual nurses appeared committed to 'felt-fairness' in terms of pay levels. In 1997, the Review Body commented that they were:

' ... *disappointed that communication by Trusts about their pay strategies often appear to be so poor*' (para 79).

5.4.1 Pay in the non-NHS sectors

The RCN membership surveys conducted by the IES normally include about 500 non-NHS nurses. These include nurses in independent hospitals, nursing and residential care homes, hospices, prisons, the military, industry and commerce. In general, employers in these sectors have tended to follow Whitley and the Review Body recommendations in setting their pay rates to roughly parallel national scales. The fact that the 1996 Review Body report made no recommendation on the size of any local pay element, meant that some employers (for example, the Prison Service) began to put new negotiating processes in place.

Given the close, if loosening, link between NHS and non-NHS nurses' pay determination, it is not surprising that the pattern of responses to the pay satisfaction statements, by nurses working outside the NHS, has broadly mirrored those of NHS nurses.

The 1997 survey shows that 58 per cent of non-NHS nurses agreed that: '*I could be paid more for less effort if I left nursing*'. This is slightly lower than the comparable value for NHS nurses (62 per cent). The proportion (22 per cent) of non-NHS nurses who agreed that: '*Considering the work I do, I am paid well*' was almost double the NHS figure (12 per cent).

However, there are important differences among these groups of non-NHS nurses. The proportion agreeing that: *'I could be paid more for less effort if I left nursing'* varies from 51 per cent for those working in GP practices to 61 per cent of nursing/residential homes, 62 per cent of agency and bank nurses and 66 per cent in independent hospitals (see Figure 5.6).

Figure 5.6 'I could be paid more for less effort if I left nursing': nurses working in nursing or residential homes, 1993, 1995 and 1997

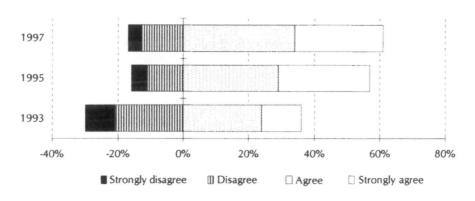

Source: Seccombe and Smith, 1997a

There are similar differences in response to the second statement: *'considering the work I do, I am paid well'*. 28 per cent of practice nurses agreed with the statement, compared with only one in ten (11 per cent) agency and bank nurses, one in six (17 per cent) independent hospital nurses and one in five (20 per cent) of nursing/residential home nurses.

Responses from nurses working in different non-NHS sectors (Figure 5.7) indicates that the majority of these in each of the four sectors agreed with the statement that they could be paid more for less effort if they left nursing. Nurses in independent hospitals were most likely to agree with the statement.

Figure 5.7 'I could be paid more for less effort if I left nursing': non-NHS nurses, by employment sector

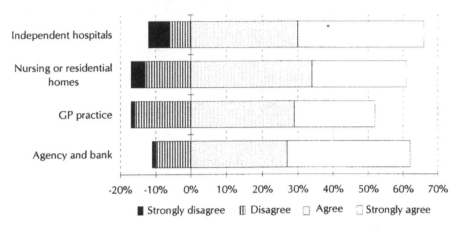

Source: Seccombe and Smith, 1997a

5.5 Summary

The period from the establishment of the Review Body in the mid 1980s, until the early 1990s, was one of comparative stability, in terms of the 'real' level of nurses' pay. More recently, the focus of pay determination has broadened to include national and local elements, but with much uncertainty about the extent to which there would be any 'real' local pay. The 1997 Review Body report, by slowing down the pace of change towards local pay, merely reflected the situation in which many NHS trusts had found themselves, that is ill-equipped to sustain such change. The end result for most NHS nurses remains a 'Whitley' based pay packet, but one determined by a more devolved (critics argue a more convoluted) and less certain process.

Research from the United States suggests that localised pay determination may not lead to the pay variations between nurses and between employing units that some have predicted. This is because of a tendency for employers who share labour markets to formally collaborate in pay determination, or informally collate pay information. This can dampen down pay variation and the pressure for pay increases.

Further constraint on local freedom will occur if the new Labour government introduces national minimum wage legislation or national 'basic' rates of pay for different groups. This is likely to lead to increased focus by local management on other elements of the employment package, and on working patterns and skill mix, as they search for methods of containing unit labour costs.

Pay has been a central element of most of the national attitudinal surveys of nurses conducted in Britain in the last decade. An examination of trends reflected by these surveys serves to highlight three major issues:

- NHS nurses have become less satisfied with their pay in recent years.

- NHS nurses are less satisfied with their pay than nurses working in other sectors.

- NHS nurses have not been convinced by arguments put forward in favour of moving from national to local pay determination.

The results of the 1996 RCN Membership survey highlighted the failure to win the hearts and minds of nurses in relation to the process of local pay determination in the NHS. The extent to which this was due to poor communication, (*ie* NHS nurses do not 'understand' the 'benefits' of local pay) or due to disagreement with the message (*ie* NHS nurses 'understand' local pay and do not regard it as a benefit) remains open to question. The election of a Labour government in 1997 has, in any case, shifted the focus away from local pay determination towards a broader human resource strategy.

6 Changing Career Patterns

6.1 Introduction

The major changes in health and social care outlined in the introduction to this book have a profound influence on the careers of nurses. In particular, the shift towards a primary health care led service and transformations in the delivery of care mean that nursing careers are becoming less predictable, less linear and more complex. Recent years have seen an erosion of the clinical hierarchy as health care providers have adopted flatter and more varied organisational structures. At the same time, there has been significant growth of clinical careers in community and primary care and in the independent and wider health care sectors.

There has been much rhetoric around careers in recent times. Some organisations have said they no longer offer careers, that the very notion of a career is dead, that there are no jobs for life anymore. The effect is a reported sense of growing insecurity and uncertainty. Individual employees who are tied to a location through family commitments or mortgages, or those who work for monopsony employers, are likely to feel more vulnerable than those who possess easily transferable skills.

The way in which careers are understood and operate is profoundly affected by the context within which they exist. This occurs on a number of different levels which can be termed social, economic and political change, organisational change and changing values and attitudes.

In terms of organisational change, the last two decades have been characterised by the following general features:

- attempts by organisations to cut costs by reducing manpower, for example the imposition in the NHS in 1996 of a 5 per cent cut in the M2 management figure (defined as staff earning more than £20,000 a year);

- the restructuring of organisations through de-layering and devolving. For example, the number of senior nurse posts has fallen by 1,300 (36 per cent) between 1989 and 1994;

- the outsourcing of some activities; paralleled in the health service by the growing use of bank and agency staff; and

- attempts to achieve greater flexibility through numerical, temporal and functional changes. In nursing, this has led to the growth of short-term contracts and changing shift patterns.

In careers terms the effect of this organisational turbulence has been to encourage a rhetoric that careers are dead; to modify traditional career paths; to produce greater employer and employee uncertainty about the future; to pressurise employees to work harder and longer hours, and to transfer more responsibility for career development to the individual.

The backdrop of key social/economic changes have included:

- A greater participation of women in the labour market. This is echoed in nursing by the rising participation rates of qualified nurses. As we saw in Chapter two, the proportion of qualified nurses working in nursing has risen from 60 per cent in 1971 (Sadler and Whitworth, 1975) to 68 per cent in 1991 (Lader, 1995). The latter also revealed that a further 16 per cent were engaged in non-nursing employment.

- Women are returning to work faster after having children. Career breaks in nursing tend to be comparatively short; Waite *et al* (1990) show that almost half the career breaks lasted less than two years and that most were taken before the age of 30.

- A rising proportion of single parent households. The proportion of nurses who are single parents increased from 6 per cent in 1992 to 7 per cent in 1996 (Seccombe and Smith, 1996).

- A rising elderly population, a decline in the value of the state pension and a rise in private health care provision (see Chapter 7). These factors may impact on nurses' career decisions by influencing when they are available for work and their mobility. A rising proportion (16 per cent in 1996) of nurses have caring responsibilities for elderly relatives or other adults (Seccombe and Smith, 1996).

Generally, there has been a decline in the labour market dominance of big employers. In the health sector, this is reflected in the rapid growth of nurses' employment in nursing and residential homes, in GP practices, community trusts and other settings. Prior to the current decade, the proportion of nurses employed outside the hospital sector changed little. Briggs (1972) showed that in 1971, less than 10 per cent of nursing staff (wte) in GB were employed in community nursing. Evidence from the 1996 RCN/IES survey showed that nearly 40 per cent of nurses were employed outside hospital settings (Seccombe and Smith, 1996). Other social and economic factors are the persistence of comparatively high unemployment and fear of redundancy. These may act to dampen turnover and wastage from nursing jobs which may appear comparatively secure.

To summarise, these factors mean that there is a more varied, but better educated, workforce with more complex domestic responsibilities, often working in smaller organisations and in times of greater job insecurity. Seccombe and Smith (1996) found that only 16 per cent of NHS nurses agreed with the statement *'Nursing will continue to offer me a secure job for several years'*. Only four years earlier, over half (52 per cent) of the survey respondents had agreed with the same statement (Seccombe, Ball & Patch, 1993). For individual nurses then, there is greater need for careers which enable them to balance domestic and work roles in an environment of uncertainty.

Political changes have also impacted on careers. Some policies have acted to exacerbate feelings of insecurity, while others may have coincided with attitudinal and social changes. Since 1979, successive Conservative governments pursued policies which emphasised:

- Deregulation of the economy. In the health service context this was manifested in the introduction of the internal market by which purchaser/provider service contracts were negotiated on an annual basis.

- Privatisation and market exposure of public services (*eg* via contracting out and the Private Finance Initiative).

- Individualism rather than collectivism (*eg* trade union reform).

- Reduced government intervention (*eg* local pay bargaining), greater employer (*eg* statutory sick pay) or employee responsibility (*eg* pensions).

- Market incentives: profit and performance related pay, local pay bargaining (see Chapter 5).

More generally, there have been shifts in social values and attitudes which have undermined employers' old paternalistic model of careers. These changes, which include, for example, the growing desire of individuals to be better informed, to have a more inclusive and less deferential relationship with employers, are coupled with continuing support for social protection and a search for a higher quality of life.

In the remainder of this chapter we explore changing career patterns and report on trends in nurses' career satisfaction and career progression.

6.2 The traditional nursing career

In reality, nurses' careers have always been varied and individualistic. Nevertheless, there was a dominant model of careers, in general, which prevailed until comparatively recently. In this model, a series of jobs provided the potential for a steady progression of salary and responsibility until relatively late in life. From this career plateau the individual would retire. In this 'typical' career, there would be a number of job moves, but with most of the career being spent in one organisation. In this model 'careers' happened almost mechanistically, and followed a strongly delineated path with well defined steps.

In nursing, however, this model has not held true for many individuals - the reality comprised far fewer promotional moves and far more discontinuity. As Celia Davies, writing in the *Collapse of the Conventional Career,* argues ' ... *nursing reflects conventional career thinking and values conventional careers in a context where such careers have always been impossible for many of those involved'* (Davies, 1990).

Hockey (1976) identified three career types based on a study of 586 Scottish nurses' work histories. These were:

- the stable career — showing no breaks of three months or more;

- the dual career — a moderately stable career interrupted by breaks of more than three months but less than three years; and

- the interrupted career — breaks in service of more than three years.

Just under a third of nurses fell into the interrupted career group with 16 per cent in the dual career category. Over half the staff nurses and midwives fell into the interrupted career group, compared to only 17 per cent of sisters/teachers and 14 per cent of nurse administrators. The study also found that 59 per cent of staff nurses worked part-time compared with 13 per cent of sisters/teachers and less than 1 per cent of administrators. The Hockey study, conducted two decades ago, clearly showed that a high proportion of nurses married in their early twenties, left employment to have children in their late twenties and returned to nursing, on a part-time basis, in their early thirties. Those that followed this path were less likely to progress upwards than those who remained in continual employment.

In the past, most newly qualified nurses entered the workforce by taking up employment in the NHS, mainly in the NHS hospital sector. Subsequent moves (in some cases after a career break) could be to the NHS community sector or to the independent sector. However, data from some Colleges of nurse education show a sharp rise in the proportions of newly qualified nurses taking up employment in the non-NHS sector prior to joining the NHS (Yorkshire Health, 1994). Currently, much of this sector (particularly elderly care) is made up of a large number of small operators and provides little in the way of career opportunities. If, as some commentators anticipate, this market becomes increasingly dominated by fewer, larger operators, they may increasingly be able to offer longer term careers outside the NHS. Figure 6.1 illustrates this for elderly care.

Figure 6.1 Past and future career paths: nurses in elderly care

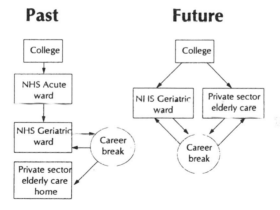

Source: IES, after Yorkshire Health, 1994

A survey of pre-registration nursing students conducted by IES in 1994 probed the extent to which students planned to work in the NHS on qualification (Seccombe, Jackson and Patch, 1995). Almost three-quarters of conventional nursing course students reported that they wanted to work in the NHS on qualification. In contrast less than two-thirds of pre-registration diploma and nursing degree course students wanted to work in the NHS. This is not because very many more students in these groups said that they did not want to work in the NHS but rather because more were undecided whether they wanted to work in the NHS or not. Nearly a third of students in these groups were undecided about their future careers.

For those students who said that they did not want to work in the NHS when they qualified, or who were undecided, by far the main concern which they expressed about working in the NHS was uncertainty about future career opportunities.

Future nursing careers are likely to be more diverse, with entry from education into a number of sectors, to be characterised by short-term contracts and multiple moves between sectors, and with nurses having shorter and later career breaks.

6.3 Clinical grading

The career structure for NHS nurses remained largely unaltered from the creation of the service in 1948 until 1988, with the notable exception of an increase in availability of promoted posts in nurse management as a result of the 'Salmon' reform. During that period it became increasingly clear that the existing career structure failed to reward clinical skills and responsibilities. As a consequence, many nurses felt that they could only progress by leaving direct patient care for nurse management.

In response to rising concern the Management and Staff sides of Nursing and Midwifery Staff Negotiating Council set up a joint working group on pay and clinical grading in 1985. The working group produced definitions for nine grades (designated A to I, lowest to highest) to replace all existing grades from nursing auxiliary up to senior nurse (grade 7). The 1988 Review Body then produced a pay spine for the new structure.

Clinical grading was not implemented without difficulty (see Chapter 5), but did represent a major boost for 'promoted' posts within NHS clinical nursing. However, since its implementation, managerial reorganisation and cost containment have served to reduce the career opportunities instigated in 1988/99.

The major changes in grade distribution in the structure since 1989 have been a drop of 11.4 per cent in the number of G grade posts and a 41.5 per cent drop in the number of I grade posts. Clinical nurses are now concentrated in the three main clinical grades (D, E and F) which have has risen from 63 per cent to 70 per cent of the total (Pay Review Body, 1992).

Progression through the clinical grading structure has slowed since its introduction. Table 6.1 compares the clinical grade five years after first

Table 6.1 Clinical grades of first level registered nurses working in the NHS in their fifth year after first registering (per cent)

Grade after five years:	Year first registered:				
	1989	1990	1991	1992	1993
D	21.3	21.3	31.5	44.4	45.2
E	71.9	60.6	64.0	49.2	51.6
F	4.5	3.2	2.7	2.4	2.2
G	2.2	1.1	1.8	3.2	–
H	–	–	–	0.8	1.1
Base number	*89*	*94*	*111*	*124*	*93*

Source: Seccombe and Smith, 1997a

registration for successive cohorts of nurses who first registered since the introduction of clinical grading.

We can see from the table that by 1993, nearly three-quarters (71.9 per cent) of the 1989 cohort were graded E and 21.3 per cent were graded D. In contrast, by 1997, only half (51.6 per cent) of those who first registered in 1993 were graded E and 45.2 per cent were graded D.

As nurse management structures have 'flattened' in the 1990s, career structures and career opportunities for clinical nurses have changed (Ball *et al*, 1995) and the need to consider new ways of sustaining career development within clinical practice has arisen. The existing NHS clinical grading structure has been seen by some as overly mechanistic and too rigidly focused on managerial and resource issues, rather than on clinical excellence (see Buchan, 1992).

Increased patient throughput, higher levels of patient acuity and changes in the deployment and roles of junior doctors, are recognised as making clinical nursing a more demanding job with new and complex responsibilities. These provide additional pressure for career structures which more explicitly recognise the value of nurses' work in delivering patient care. Linked to this is the belief that job satisfaction can be enhanced by linking pay and career progression to the attainment of advanced clinical skills and expertise, reinforced by continuing professional development.

Options being considered by some in the NHS include the introduction of skills or competency-based pay or clinical ladders. A clinical ladder is a grading structure which facilitates career progression, and associated pay differentiation, by defining different levels of clinical and professional practice in nursing. Progression is dependent on the individual meeting defined criteria of clinical excellence, skills and competence, professional expertise and educational attainment (Buchan, 1997). It differs from the existing NHS clinical grading structure in that it is individualised and places emphasis on the continual development, appraisal and competence of the individual, rather than the post they occupy.

The introduction of skills or competency based pay or of clinical ladders would require a significant cultural change in NHS nursing. The focus on the individual nurse, and on progression through individual application, has not been the norm in the NHS, where national grading and incremental progression has been the convention. NHS nurses have become familiar, over the last five decades, with a standard national template for pay and grading. The introduction of career ladders would mean that like-for-like inter-organisation job mobility is no longer the norm, and would put greater emphasis on an individual's portfolio of skills, qualifications and competencies.

6.4 Career progression

The Briggs report (1972) found that nurses were very cautious about career progression. More than half the nurses surveyed were reported to be 'happy' to stay in their current grades and were not looking for promotion. This response is in marked contrast to that of the 1996 IES/RCN survey in which more than two-thirds of NHS nurses agreed with the statement '*I am interested in career progression*'.

Both Briggs (1972) and IES (1996) asked hospital based nurses what they expected to be doing in two years time. Table 6.2 compares the responses of staff nurses (full-time and part-time) in both surveys. Although the response categories are not precisely the same, useful comparisons can be made.

There are two significant points of comparison between these surveys which tend to bear out the changing view of nursing careers outlined earlier. Firstly, nurses are now less optimistic about their promotion prospects (25 per cent expect to be in a higher grade in two years time compared with 31 per cent in 1972). Secondly, more expect to work outside nursing (8 per cent compared with 4 per cent in 1972).

Briggs also reported that two-thirds of community nurses and half the hospital nurses believed that their career prospects were 'not very good'. In

Table 6.2 Comparison of anticipated employment in two years, 1972 and 1996 surveys

	Full-time		Part-time	
	1972	1996	1972	1996
Same job	22%	35%	56%	55%
Similar job in another unit	13%	19%	8%	13%
Higher grade	31%	25%	7%	8%
Local Authority nursing	6%	-	4%	-
Another nursing job	13%	-	7%	-
Non-NHS nursing	-	4%	-	6%
Non-nursing job	4%	8%	1%	6%
Not working	9%	4%	14%	6%
Other	-	3%	-	2%
Don't know	2%	1%	2%	2%
Missing		1%		2%
Base number	508	732	585	428

Source: Briggs, 1972 & Seccombe and Smith, 1996

comparison, the 1996 IES/RCN survey found that 67 per cent of community and 70 per cent of hospital based nurses agreed with the statement '*It will be difficult for me to progress from my current grade.*'

The extent to which nurses expect to progress is also related to their current grade. Those in D and F grades were most optimistic about grade progression, but even in these grades, 61 per cent and 67 per cent respectively, agreed with the statement that: '*it would be difficult to achieve career progression*'. Almost three-quarters (73 per cent) of E grades and 77 per cent of H grades agreed with the statement. Least optimistic were enrolled nurses, 72 per cent of whom agreed that it would be difficult for them to progress (in part this may reflect the higher proportion of enrolled nurses who work part-time).

6.5 Career satisfaction

In the IES/RCN series of surveys, nurses have been asked to rate their satisfaction with five aspects of their careers. These statements are:

- *'I have a considerable say in the way my career develops.'*
- *'I don't know where my career in nursing is going.'*
- *'There is open dialogue about my career with my manager.'*
- *'I am in a dead end job.'* *(scoring reversed)*
- *'I have a good chance to get ahead in nursing.'*

Figure 6.2 summarises the responses of NHS and non-NHS nurses to these items and reveals important differences between the two groups. On almost all these items, non-NHS nurses are more satisfied than their NHS counterparts. For example, over half the non-NHS nurses agree that they can determine the way their career develops, compared with two-fifths (42 per cent) of NHS nurses. Over 40 per cent of NHS nurses say that they do not know where their nursing careers are going and only 37 per cent say that they have an open dialogue about their career with their manager. The latter compares with over two-fifths of non-NHS nurses.

Figure 6.2 NHS and non-NHS nurses career satisfaction, 1997

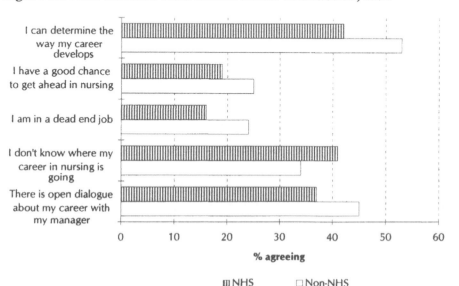

Source: IES/1997 RCN Membership Survey

Only a fifth (19 per cent) of NHS nurses (25 per cent of the non-NHS) agreed that they had a good chance to '*get ahead in nursing*', a view which seems to accord with the lack of grade progression identified earlier. Despite this, few nurses (16 per cent in the NHS, 24 per cent in the non-NHS) believe that they are in a dead end job.

6.6 Working abroad

Nurses who are registered in the UK have a further career option. They can choose to make use of their nursing qualifications by working in countries other than the UK. There has been periodic debate about the extent to which the numbers of UK nurses moving abroad represents a drain on resources, but from the point of view of individuals, there can be a number of attractions to working overseas. This section examines the 'outflow' of nursing from the UK, and the reasons for that outflow.

The UKCC register can be used to examine trends in outflow and to assist in identifying major 'destination' countries. Verification documents are issued by the UKCC to regulatory bodies in other countries in respect of UK based nurses applying to nurse there. However, there are limitations to using the UKCC data to estimate outflow. Firstly, verification indicates intent, rather than the actuality of working as a nurse overseas. Secondly, application for verification may occur some time after the geographical move to the other country has occurred. Thirdly, more than one verification may be issued in respect of an individual nurse, so there may be some double counting. Having noted these limitations, the UKCC data is never the less the best available source of information on trends in the magnitude of outflow of nurses from the UK, and in identifying the main destination for nurses leaving, or considering leaving the UK.

Figure 6.3 illustrates the overall trend in verifications issued on an annual basis since 1984/85. The number of verifications issued for the major 'destination' countries are also illustrated. The number of verifications issued annually increased over the 1980s, to peak at 8,626 in 1990/91 and has since declined, to 3,056 in 1994/95, rising to 3,607 in 1995/96. This represents a marked decline, by more than half, over the period. An examination of international nurse mobility (Buchan, Seccombe and Ball, 1992) predicted that there would be a decline in the number of UK based nurses emigrating to North America and Australasia, as budgetary cuts and healthcare reforms in those countries reduced the demand for recruitment from abroad. The extent to which this has occurred

Figure 6.3　Verification documents issued by the UKCC, 1984/85 to 1995/96

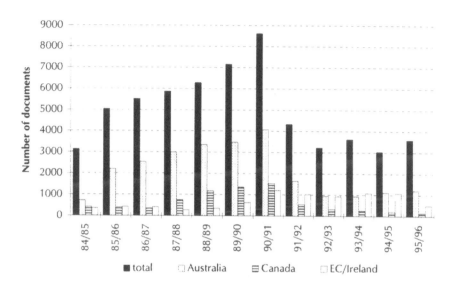

Source: UKCC Statistical analysis of the Council's Professional Register

is best illustrated by the example of Australia, for which the number of verifications issued in 1995/96 is at a level of only one quarter of the number issued five years earlier.

With the exception of Eire, European countries are not favoured destinations for UK nurses, even with free mobility legislation in place. In 1990/91 the countries of the EU accounted for 14 per cent of verifications issued by the UKCC. In 1992/93 this figure had risen to 29 per cent of all verifications, but by 1995/96 it had fallen back again, to 14 per cent of the total. The overall pattern of verifications issued indicates that outflow to the English speaking countries of Australasia and North America has declined but continues to be more significant than to other countries.

The total of 3,607 verifications issued in 1995/96 represented a small potential annual 'outflow', compared to the number of practitioners on the UKCC register. Whilst this may not be regarded as significant in numerical terms, it is similar to the number of new entrants to the Register in that year, from Scotland, Wales and Northern Ireland combined. It should also be stressed that there do appear to be international 'shortages' of particular specialties, such as intensive care nurses and theatre/OR nurses. The UKCC data cannot be used for an investigation of the extent to which the UK may be 'losing' hard-to-replace nursing skills to other countries, but it is apparent from advertisements in the UK nursing press that many agencies recruiting for work abroad are active in these 'shortage' specialties.

Information from two of the annual surveys of RCN members gives more information on the motivations of UK nurses who have previously worked abroad. The survey conducted in 1992 found that one in ten respondents had held a nursing job outside the UK, and that this figure was much higher amongst non-NHS nurses (Buchan, Seccombe, Ball, 1992).

A more detailed survey (n=4,000 nurses) of RCN members conducted in 1994 identified 251 nurses (6 per cent) who had at some time worked as a nurse outside the UK (Buchan, Seccombe, Thomas, 1997). The study examined the biographical profile and career histories of this sample of 251 qualified nurses who had trained in the UK, but had since nursed in a country other than the UK, and examined their reasons for nursing abroad. The study confirmed the findings of previous research that 'returners' from abroad were more likely to work in non-NHS nursing than to be employed by the NHS. One in seven (17%) of non-NHS nurses reported having had a nursing job outside the UK, compared to 7 per cent among NHS nurses.

The survey found that over seventy countries were reported as having been the location for nursing abroad. More than a third (37 per cent) of these nurses reported that they had worked in more than one country. Australia, Canada, Saudi Arabia, Germany and the US were the most commonly reported countries. The reported length of time spent nursing abroad ranged from two months to nineteen years per visit.

One of the key areas examined in the survey was the motivation of those nurses who had worked abroad. When asked to indicate the main reason for nursing abroad the most common reason (28 per cent) was to gain non-UK nursing experience. There were also 'non professional' reasons for moving country. One quarter (24 per cent) of respondents reported that their main reason for nursing abroad was that they moved with their partner/family. Combining travel and work is a third motivation for working abroad. One in six respondents (16 per cent) reported that their reason for nursing abroad was as a working holiday - mainly to North America and Australia. The desire to improve economic status and financial security is a fourth major motivation for migrants. Financial reasons were given by 14 per cent of respondents as the main reason for nursing abroad - countries of the Middle East were prominent in this outflow.

Other main reasons for nursing abroad given by respondents included voluntary/aid work (6 per cent) mainly in Africa, Middle East and Asia; to gain a non-UK nursing qualification (2 per cent), and study tour (1 per cent). A small, but significant proportion, of those who reported nursing abroad were nurses who had worked with the British Armed Forces in Germany, Cyprus, Gibraltar, Hong Kong and the countries directly affected during the Gulf War.

The survey also examined the opinions of nurses who had worked abroad as to where it was easiest to get a nursing job on returning to the UK. The area perceived to be easiest to get nursing work reported by respondents was agency nursing, with 86 per cent reporting that in their opinion it was 'very easy' or 'easy' to get work in this area. The independent sector, particularly nursing homes, was also regarded as comparatively easy to enter.

In contrast, the NHS was not regarded as an easy source of employment by these nurses. More than half of respondents felt that it was 'difficult or very difficult' to get a job in NHS nursing on returning from nursing abroad. Of those respondents who reported that in their opinion it was 'difficult' to get a job in NHS nursing, half (49 per cent) were currently working in non-NHS nursing, with 5 per cent currently working in GP practice nursing and a further 5 per cent currently working in non-nursing employment.

The requirement for language capabilities to communicate with clients and patients is likely to act as a barrier to many nurses who might be considering working abroad. This also helps explain the main outflows to the English speaking countries of North America, Australia and New Zealand. The survey conducted in 1992 (Buchan, Seccombe, Ball, 1992) found that only 18 per cent of UK nurses claimed to have a working knowledge of a non English language.

6.7 Summary

This chapter has outlined the effects of changing organisational, social and political contexts on nursing careers. This discussion has emphasised that nursing careers are becoming less structured, less predictable and more complex, changes which induce an obvious sense of insecurity, uncertainty and confusion. The key points made in the chapter are that:

- the clinical grading hierarchy has been eroded since its establishment in 1988/89; there are now significantly fewer posts at G and I grades;

- a cohort analysis demonstrates a 'slow down' in recent years of progression through the clinical grading scale;

- in response, a majority of NHS nurses feel that it will be difficult for them to progress, in terms of their clinical grades;

- at the same time, a higher proportion of nurses reveal themselves to be interested in career progression than was the case twenty-five years ago;

- a high proportion (40 per cent) of NHS nurses say that they don't know where their nursing careers are going and little more than a third have an open dialogue about their careers with their manager;

- there has been a clear measurable decline in the level of nurses' career satisfaction since the early 1990s; and

- working abroad is a career route used only by a minority of UK nurses.

7 Workforce Planning in Nursing

Planning the size of the nursing workforce is a serious and complex business. Pre-registration nurse education costs in excess of £35,000[10] for each new nurse. Over-estimating the demand for newly qualified nurses by even a small percentage would have substantial financial implications as well as having the potential to raise nurse unemployment, whilst under-estimating demand would have enormous costs in terms of the volume and quality of service provided and the workloads imposed on staff.

As decision making is further devolved, with the creation of NHS trusts, local Education and Training Consortia (ETCs) in England and the growing significance of the non-NHS labour market, establishing an independent national overview of the nursing workforce is an increasingly complex task.

Since the early 1940s, successive governments have sought to plan the labour market for doctors. They have attempted this by forecasting the demand for doctors and adjusting the supply (medical school intake) accordingly. Medical workforce planning has been a highly centralised activity undertaken by a series of *ad hoc* committees (Goodenough in 1944, Willink in 1957), Royal Commissions (Todd, 1968) and, since July 1991, a standing advisory committee (Medical Manpower Standing Advisory Committee). These committees have directly advised the Secretary of State for Health on the future numbers of doctors and required intakes to medical schools.

In contrast, central government has continued to consider it both impractical and inappropriate to plan the demand and supply of nurses nationally at a UK level (although Scotland has retained and developed a national mechanism). Any work which has been done has tended to be piecemeal and devolved, focusing on monitoring numbers and managing costs, rather than considering roles, skills and competencies, participation rates and incentives.

Proceeding along separate lines in this way implies that any substitution possibilities, between the work of doctors and nurses, are limited. One recent review (Richardson and Maynard, 1995) suggests that substitution possibilities of doctors' work are important, although their cost-effectiveness has been under-evaluated. In these circumstances it seems inappropriate to continue making decisions about nurse numbers in isolation from future decisions about numbers of doctors and others.

Even given an assumption that the ratio between different staffing inputs are fixed, the implications of 'medical' workforce forecasting have been largely ignored by workforce planners dealing with other staff. MWSAC's[11] second report recommended that the number of medical students be increased annually to a maximum target of 4,970 by the year 2000 (with total doctor numbers projected to rise to 126,500 by the year 2010). This seems to have had no explicit place in considerations to determine the size of intakes to pre-registration nursing over the same period.

This view is now changing. In a memorandum to the Commons Health Committee, The Department of Health *'recognises the need for better integration of medical and non-medical workforce planning'* as a result of moves towards multi-disciplinary team working and the blurring of traditional roles (Department of Health, 1996c). The need to integrate workforce planning was also given prominence in EL (96)45 *Priorities and Planning Guidance for the NHS: 1997/98* which includes the development of integrated workforce planning as one of its priority actions. Many recent policy changes have implicitly assumed that nurses will take on more responsibilities (*eg* the reduction in junior doctors' hours). The development of the nurse practitioner and the Primary Care Act, also highlight the need for a unified national overview.

7.1 Recent history

Until recently, there has been surprisingly little attempt to maintain a national overview of the nursing workforce, or to undertake nurse supply planning, at a national level in the UK. What is not surprising is that the work that has been done has tended to focus narrowly on counting heads and whole time equivalents, rather than taking into account skill requirements, participation rates or incentives.

In the 1970s and 1980s the Department of Health and Social Security (DHSS) delegated responsibility for planning nurse numbers to health authorities as part of their overall strategic planning role. At this time the emphasis was on monitoring the numbers in employment, with central control on numbers exercised only through limiting overall expenditure by health authorities.

The absence of a national nurse workforce planning strategy for nurses was highlighted by the Briggs Committee in its 1972 report, and by the 1979 Royal Commission on the NHS. From 1979, the DHSS sought to monitor health authorities' demand for nurses through the strategic planning exercise. However, a survey conducted in 1979 showed that the scope and quality of manpower planning varied greatly between regions (Long and Mercer, 1981). The National Audit Office (NAO) subsequently concluded that *'these plans were of little use as the manpower content was limited and compiled on an inconsistent basis between regions. The strategic plans based the future demand for nurses more on financial projections than on likely service developments'* (NAO, 1985).

In its 1985 report the NAO criticised the lack of reliable information by which the health departments and health authorities could monitor and control nursing staff numbers. The NAO also criticised the lack of guidance given to health authorities on methodologies to be used. The NAO study observed that some authorities set nursing establishments on the basis of affordability rather than need.

Research on national level nurse workforce planning was undertaken in the mid-1980s, in relation to proposed changes to nurse education. The RCN's Commission on Education (RCN, 1985) commissioned the Institute of Manpower Studies (IMS) to assess the manpower implications of moving to a single level of basic qualification and changes in student status. IMS developed a national model which could be used to project nurse training requirements in England (Hutt *et al*, 1985). The UKCC also commissioned work to examine the workforce implications of Project 2000 (Price Waterhouse, 1987). At the same time, the projected decline in the number of 18 year olds was fuelling fears of a potential shortfall in recruits to nursing (Conroy and Stidston, 1988).

7.2 Working Paper 10 — Education and training

The NHS reforms held up the possibility that the costs of non-medical education and training could put trusts and other healthcare providers at a cost and price disadvantage when competing for contracts. It was felt important to remove these costs from pricing decisions in order to maintain an adequate supply of key professional and technical skills.

At the time it was also felt that the wide range of organisations involved in the funding, planning and provision of education and training needed to be rationalised.

Working Paper 10 was one of a series of papers produced by the Department of Health following the Review of the NHS. These papers described in detail how particular proposals in the White Paper 'Working for Patients' would be implemented. Working Paper 10 was concerned with the implications of the reform for education and training (Department of Health, 1989). It recognised a number of practical problems in establishing a system for assessing manpower demand. These included:

- an expected increase in the number of employers of healthcare professionals;

- an anticipated growth in demand from non-NHS employers;

- the possibility that employers would inflate demand for newly-qualified staff — in part because some of the training costs would be directly funded and also because employers would base estimates of future demand on expectations about winning contracts which may not be secured; and

- a conflict of interest for DHAs seeking manpower information from providers who may be competing for contracts from that purchaser.

Working Paper 10 gave responsibility for identifying demand to Regional Health Authorities (RHAs). Each RHA would therefore be responsible for setting up mechanisms to ensure that manpower information was collected from employers and that manpower demand was assessed. It was intended that regions become 'self-sufficient' whilst recognising that the unequal distribution of training facilities would necessitate inter-Regional co-operation.

Under the Working Paper 10 arrangements, Regions were responsible for identifying employer demand (both NHS and others) for newly qualified staff so that sufficient funds could be earmarked to ensure the supply of training places. They then commissioned the education and training places required.

Workforce planning to determine the number of places was largely based on the collection of unit level workforce plans, generally via proforma returned to the region. Regions would then scrutinise these returns for internal and external consistency. The plans of individual units were then aggregated at regional level to form the basis for contracts with education providers.

The NHS Management Executive would then monitor the aggregate training decisions of RHAs to ensure that collective under (or over) training would not occur. In 1994, for example, it instructed Regions to increase the number of places commissioned for pre-registration nurse education and training by 5 per cent.

7.3 The National Balance Sheet Exercise

In 1991 the NHS introduced a new mechanism to monitor regional Working Paper 10 staffing requirements. The purpose of this, the National Balance Sheet Exercise, was to *'ensure that regions are making a fair contribution to the education and training of staff groups covered . . .* ' [12]. The purpose was therefore, to meet both local demand as well as ensuring that the national supply was not undermined by local decisions.

The exercise was service led, in that Regional Health Authorities aggregated the workforce plans of NHS and other healthcare providers, to give an overall estimate of demand for education places. The Balance Sheet Exercise consisted of an annual survey of employing units, collecting data on the number of whole time equivalent staff in post, a five year projected growth of staff in post and a five year projected demand for newly qualified staff.

A set of indicators (so-called traffic lights) were produced to monitor the effects of regional plans on national supply. For most nurses these indicators (training commissions divided by demand for newly qualified staff) were set at the following levels:

Red   <110%   Numbers entering training are insufficient to meet demand after attrition and retention are taken into account.

Amber   111-124%   Numbers entering training should be sufficient to meet demand after allowing for attrition and retention.

Green   >124%   Numbers entering training appear too high, safe to consider reducing intakes.

If the indicator for a particular staff group in one Region was green, but nationally the figure was red, then that Region should not cut its commissions unless compensating increases were made in other regions.

In practice the Balance Sheet Exercise faced a number of problems. These included:

- Few employers had (or have) reliable historic data on wastage upon which to base projections. As a result, short-term trends (which have been influenced by general economic recession) tended to be more influential. Employers with higher than average wastage tended to assume that they would improve retention; those with lower than average wastage continued to forecast low levels.

- Some employers may have built into their plans assumptions about skill mix which have not been realised (see Buchan, Seccombe and Ball, 1996).

- The short-term nature of service contracting made it difficult to project future workforce requirements over a sufficient period. Demand for newly qualified nurses was therefore more likely to be based on current vacancy levels and wastage assumptions.

- Variable training routes and course lengths were not properly accounted for — at least in the initial Balance Sheet Exercises.

- Some non-NHS employers were unwilling, or unable, to take part in the exercise.

As we saw in Chapter Two, the intakes to pre-registration nurse education, determined as a result of this exercise fell in subsequent years despite apparently rising demand for nursing care. There are several reasons for this anomaly. These include:

- Prior to the introduction of Project 2000, hospital employers had an incentive (*ie* access to a comparatively cheap labour supply) to keep student numbers high. Project 2000 introduced supernumerary status for pre-registration nursing students and reduced their workforce contribution.

- The traditional nurse education system also encouraged employers to guarantee employment to these students on qualification, rather than to recruit more expensive returners from the pool.

- Demand for newly qualified nurses in the NHS hospital sector is now more likely to be based on the actual level of D grade vacancies — until recently these vacancy levels may have been depressed by comparatively low turnover and wastage and by enrolled nurse conversion.

- In contrast NHS community units have traditionally sought to recruit experienced nurses from the pool into District Nursing and Health

Visiting. As a result they too tend not to identify demand for newly qualified nurses.

- The rapid and largely unanticipated growth of employment in GP practice and independent sector nursing has been fed from the now depleted pool of returners, reducing the scope for NHS recruitment from this source.

In addition to this bottom up approach to determining the size of intakes to education, the Department of Health commissioned a national workforce modelling project in 1995 and in 1996 to examine the longer term demand for registered nurses, and to convert this into a demand figure for newly qualified staff. This top-down approach, which uses participation rate modelling, was intended to provide a check on the outcomes of the bottom-up exercise. The results of these exercises have not been made public and it is therefore not possible to assess the implications of this work.

7.4 The new arrangements for purchasing nurse education

With the abolition of RHAs following the NHS Functions and Manpower Review, responsibility for education commissioning moved to the new NHS Executive Regional Offices. This led (in April 1996) to the creation of a new framework for education commissioning (in England) via Education and Training Consortia (ETCs) and Regional Education and Development Groups (REDGs)[13].

Education and Training Consortia had been foreshadowed in Working Paper 10 as a longer term aim. The notion that commissioning should be done by consortia of employers was put forward then for two main reasons: the number of schools of nursing was reducing, with most serving as the source of supply of new recruits to several employing units; no single trust was likely to employ the whole output of a school nor to provide the full range of clinical placements required during training.

The new arrangements are intended to give purchasers and employers (including non-NHS providers) greater responsibility for planning and commissioning non-medical education and training.

ETCs are geographically based groups (between four and eight in each NHS Region in England) of healthcare purchasers, NHS providers, GPs and non-NHS providers. Their principle role is to collate workforce plans, to determine demand for non-medical education places and to commission such places from education providers.

More than 40 consortia have been established in England (Scotland has retained a national mechanism with local employer input). Each has a lead organisation responsible for employing staff and co-ordinating activity. Ultimately the lead organisation will also manage the education and training budgets.

The membership composition and organisational structure of the consortia vary. Figure 7.1 shows one consortium membership.

Figure 7.1 An example of a core consortium membership

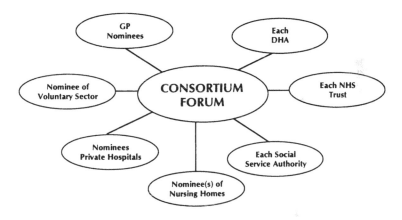

Source: Moore, 1996

In practice some consortia have faced difficulties in getting representation from all of these groups (particularly General Practitioners). Typically, the consortia are organised into a number of sub-groups along education lines (*eg* pre-registration nursing, pre-registration paramedical, post-registration, management development). In other cases, sub-groups are organised around functions (*eg* professional advisory group; workforce planning group, finance group). There may also be *ad hoc* focus groups (*eg* cancer initiative) to pick up on national priorities and ensure that these are covered (Figure 7.2).

The principle functions of the ETCs are:

- to prepare profession specific workforce profile reports;

- to collate workforce plans prepared by NHS constituent members with the determination of demand for staff from the wider health care sector;

Figure 7.3 An example of a consortium structure

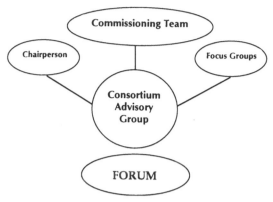

Source: Moore, 1996

- to use this information to calculate the consortium's commissioning requirements to meet service needs for newly qualified staff;

- to commission non-medical education and training direct from education providers; and

- to monitor, review and negotiate education contracts for which the consortium is responsible, in order to ensure that service needs for qualified staff are met. This will ultimately enable them to influence admission policies, educational development, quality and fitness for purpose.

Eventually, ETCs will also be charged with providing advice to the REDGs on the numbers and types of doctors required and to advise on local arrangements for post graduate medical education. It should be noted that some of these functions (*eg* commissioning places from education providers) will remain with the NHS Executive Regional Offices until ETCs are equipped to take them on.

By the end of March 1997 consortia were expected to have drawn up short, medium and long-term education and training plans and be in a position to negotiate contracts as they come up for renewal. The December 1996 primary care white paper (Primary Care: Delivering the Future) expanded the responsibility of ETCs to include the needs of practice nurses. The aim was to ensure that all consortia would (from April 1998) address the development needs of practice nurses in their investment plans.

The difficulties faced by consortia in turning workforce plans into an expression of demand, and ultimately into student intakes, are no different to those which vexed the Balance Sheet Exercise.

A number of additional concerns have also been voiced. These include:

- getting NHS trusts to share 'commercially sensitive' information about labour demand with their competitors and with their purchasers. This concern may reduce if the Labour government elected in 1997 is successful in supporting greater collaboration between trusts;

- involving the smaller non-NHS employers;

- giving sufficient weight to the activities of General Practitioners - implied by a primary-care led NHS;

- the comparatively long education planning cycles (five years) compared with the short-term contracting cycles for health commissioning. Again, the new government, in its attempts to reduce the effects of the internal market and lengthen the planning cycle, may negate the impact of this factor; and

- the need to co-ordinate the plans of consortia which share labour markets — in some cases two or more ETCs may work together.

REDGs comprise representatives of each consortium within a region together with NHS Executive Regional Office representatives. Their role is to advise on the acceptability of the consortia plans. Where REDGs and ETCs disagree, the NHS Executive Regional Office has the authority to intervene.

It will be some time before these new arrangements can be properly evaluated and it remains to be seen whether they can actually overcome the problems which have affected the Balance Sheet Exercise.

7.5 Summary

Nurse supply and demand will never be perfectly matched. In any case, this is not the objective of workforce planning. The more realistic aim is to intervene when required to make any imbalance manageable and to help employers identify appropriate recruitment, retention and development strategies for dealing with the imperfections of the nursing labour market. It can also give early warning of regional or national imbalances, and provide a systematic way of correcting for previous over- or under-supply of staff.

As such, workforce planning can provide a useful aid to policy makers taking decisions about intakes to education, recruitment and retention. However, such exercises have major limitations. They do not forecast the future. Rather, they set out the implications of assumptions about future developments which tend to be based on observations of past behaviour. The value of such exercises depends crucially on the quality of the data upon which they are based, as well as the validity of the assumptions used.

The 1980s saw a lot of effort being put into counting nurses and other NHS staff and putting them in 'boxes'. Nationally, our ability to do this has probably deteriorated in recent years, rather than improved. As trusts are obliged to make fewer statutory returns to the centre, the NHS reforms have made detailed standardised aggregation of local workforce data more problematic. This places greater emphasis on the need to maintain an aggregate national overview of trends in NHS and non-NHS nurse employment.

Most importantly, whilst counting the number of nurses is an important activity, the greater challenge is to investigate how the number and mix of staff actually affects healthcare system performance. This is particularly relevant given the new Labour government's emphasis on performance management in the NHS. A starting point should be to undertake relevant regional and national supply/demand forecasting which is based on relevant assumptions. These assumptions should be derived from deliberations and informed debate of the relevant professional, employer and educational institutions, as happens in the medical staffing context.

8 Future Trends in the UK Nursing Labour Market

8.1 Introduction

The preceding chapters of this book have established the current profile of the UK nursing labour market and have identified key trends in the characteristics and employment behaviour of registered nurses. This chapter takes a forward look. The likely effect of defined changes in various facets of nurse supply and demand are analysed in relation to the level of intakes to pre-registration nurse education over the next twenty years or so. The chapter presents the results of a series of 'what if' analyses, using simulation modelling to project the numbers of nurses in the workforce over time[14]. The modelling approach taken is outlined in Appendix 3.

This modelling exercise is, of necessity, very crude. It does not, for example, attempt to examine each area of practice or each nursing specialty separately. It also does not take account of the possibility of substituting nursing staff with other healthcare workers. Nor does it attempt to integrate with medical workforce planning. All these factors have a validity which requires their consideration in the 'real' world. The reason is simple: there is not enough robust data on which to base such projections.

Simulation modelling is one technique for looking into the future to identify, and quantify, the outcomes of alternative policies (or combinations of policies) and the effects of external events. The contribution of such modelling is not to forecast the future — change and uncertainty deny us that — rather it is an exploratory process which can help to identify potential supply-demand imbalance and inform decision making. The intention of the chapter is to collate and summarise the results of these varying 'what if' scenarios; it does not and cannot, forecast what *will* happen.

8.2 Future demand for registered nurses

A persistently intractable problem affecting workforce planning in healthcare provision is that of assessing future healthcare demand. There are at least four potential influences on the level of healthcare demand over the next twenty years. These are: demography, morbidity, technology and expectations (*eg* the Patient's Charter). Some of these influences are examined briefly below.

The main demographic trend projected for the next two decades is an increase in the numbers of elderly people, particularly the very old (85 and over). Hanson *et al* (1997) have recently demonstrated that the elderly receive the largest expenditure per capita in both the Health & Community Health Services (HCHS) and Family Health Services (FHS) sectors. They estimate that over the period 1994 to 2014 the NHS will require an additional 8.25 per cent growth in real expenditure simply to cope with demographic change.

Dunnell's (1995) analysis of data from the General Household Survey shows a modest increase in self-reported morbidity over the 1980s. It is unclear whether the growing elderly population will also experience extended levels of morbidity with increasing lifespan although one review (Bone 1995) suggests a higher incidence of light to moderate disabilities (and fewer severe disabilities).

Technological change is likely to impact on demand for staffing by extending the range of treatments or quality of outcomes: it has the potential to raise the number of people who may benefit from interventions. Changes in technology are one factor contributing to rising public expectations from healthcare and an increase in expressed demand.

Historically, the use of demand estimation techniques has been only dimly acknowledged by top down measures such as norms or ratios. Implicit in such an approach is the assumption that norms remain constant, but we know that the factors affecting them such as deployment, utilisation and technology, are constantly changing. Furthermore, they assume that current staffing levels provide an acceptable standard, an assumption which is rarely tested against any objective criteria.

Demand for nursing staff is not an issue examined directly in this book and we have to put such concerns to one side. Our focus is primarily with evaluating potential variations in the supply of nurses. However, decisions about the level of intakes to pre-registration nurse education are highly sensitive to the projected level of growth in demand for registered nurses: a projection which is increasingly uncertain beyond a short horizon. Given the long lead times involved in planning intakes (*ie* the number who qualify is determined four to five years in advance), it can take even longer to correct any emerging surplus or shortfall.

Forecasting demand and then trying to adjust supply to meet it is clearly a high risk approach. If it becomes apparent that intakes to education do not meet emerging demand, it can take years to correct the shortfall.

In this section we first map out recent patterns of growth in the demand for nurses within each component of the labour market. We will subsequently explore the effects on intakes to pre-registration education of varying these rates of growth.

8.2.1 NHS nursing

The 1996 workforce planning figures returned by the NHS regions show the number of registered nurses in the NHS (England only) growing by 5.3 per cent (12,362) between 1994/95 and 1999/2000, with growth expected in all but one of the specialist areas.

Given the uncertainty of demand forecasts, it is perhaps not surprising to find that more than half (56 per cent) of the projected growth in registered nurse numbers is anticipated in the first year of the projection. Thereafter, forecast annual growth tails off, falling to less than 0.2 per cent by the end of the period.

Although there have been fluctuations, analysis of longer term trends suggest growth of around 2.7 per cent a year in the number of registered nurses employed by the NHS since the early 1970s. However, over the last ten years there has been little growth (averaging around 0.3 per cent a year) in NHS nursing employment. Public expenditure restraints may mean that there is likely to be limited real growth, if any, in the short term.

Despite the numbers of registered nurses remaining more or less constant in recent years, there have been significant increases in productivity, as evidenced by rising activity levels. Survey evidence suggests that some of this increased productivity has been achieved by increases in the numbers of hours actually being worked by nurses. The average number of excess hours worked (*ie* beyond contracted hours) by individual nurses in the 1996 IES/RCN survey was 5.9 hours, an increase on the average of 2.1 hours since 1995 (Seccombe and Smith, 1996). The extent to which productivity can continue to improve at this rate is doubtful. Implementation of the EU Working Time Directive would be a further constraint on the hours worked by some nurses.

Skill-mix and re-profiling exercises, given much prominence in recent years, have not actually resulted in the significant shift from registered nurses to un-registered support staff that some commentators (*eg* Dyson, 1991) envisaged. The Department of Health (1996b) estimate only 13,000 health care assistants in NHS employment. It may be that there is a supply-side constraint limiting skill mix change, which may ease as employers and colleges develop National Vocational Qualification based courses to cope with yet unmet demand from NHS trusts. However, recent survey evidence suggests that reducing length of stay, more rapid patient throughput and an increase in the volume of day-case surgery, has led to higher levels of patient dependency and, in some cases, an increased demand for registered nurse inputs (Buchan, Seccombe and Ball, 1996).

Other factors likely to act to maintain the demands for registered nurses, include the effects of the so called New Deal target (government policy that by 31 December 1996 no junior doctor should be working for more than 56 hours a week) and the Calman proposals for medical training grades, both of which are likely to reduce the input of junior medical grades.

Given these influences, our initial demand model assumes continuing growth in registered nurse employment within the NHS at its recent historic rate (0.3 per cent).

8.2.2 Independent acute hospitals and clinics

Between 1982 and 1994 there was an increase in the total private sector employment of registered nurses from 12,271 to 50,465 wte; an average annual growth rate of 6 per cent.

Private acute hospitals and clinics account for about 17 per cent of total registered nurses employment in the private sector. Much of the growth in this part of the private sector came in the early 1980s with an increase in capacity of some 200-300 new beds a year (Laing and Buisson, 1995). Overall, the number of beds in the UK, rose from 7,035 in 1981 to 11,681 in 1995, with two-thirds of this growth coming between 1981 and 1985. Since then growth has been more modest and, with increasing competition for private patients from the NHS, this pattern may continue.

Over the last five years, the rate of growth in employment for registered nurses in this sector has slowed to around 0.7 per cent a year. This is the figure used in our initial demand model.

8.2.3 Private nursing homes

The private sector nursing homes market, which employed 42,428 (wte) registered nurses (in England, March 1995) has been the fastest growing source of employment for nurses. The numbers in employment grew by more than 10 per cent a year until the early 1990s as the number of nursing home places grew from 20,000 in 1970 to 194,000 in 1994 (Laing and Buisson, 1995). This review predicts demand for another 72,000 places, by the turn of the century, simply to keep pace with demographic change — an increase of 37 per cent over five years (Laing and Buisson, 1995). Beyond then, the population aged over 85 is projected to grow more slowly, at an average of 2.7 per cent per annum.

Other factors which point to continuing strong demand in this sector include:

- high rates of female participation in paid employment, and a decline in the population aged 30-50, which will act to reduce the supply of informal carers;

- the rising proportion of home owners among the elderly population — able to fund care through the sale of their property; and

- the more rapid increase in the numbers of people aged 65-74.

Overall, for modelling purposes, we have assumed that demand for nurses in this sector may actually exceed the growth of the elderly population and will at least maintain its recent historic growth rate of around 3 per cent a year.

8.2.4 GP Practice nurses

There has also been sustained growth in the demand for registered nurses in general practice. Since the mid 1980s the number (wte) of practice nurses in Great Britain has increased more than four-fold to over 11,000. Although the rate of growth has slowed since the late 1980s, when the numbers were increasing by more than a thousand per year, numbers grew by 10 per cent in 1994-95.

Although the expansion of GP fundholding may continue to sustain growth in the sector, it is likely to be at more moderate levels. A growth rate of 3 per cent a year, in line with the growth in the elderly population, has been used in the initial baseline model.

8.2.5 Other employers

In addition, registered nurses also work for a range of other employers. The largest of these other employment sectors is agency nursing which employs 5,930 wte (this figure is for England only). Other employers include: the armed forces, the police, the prison service, occupational health nursing (private industry) and the voluntary sector. Gauging the overall number of nurses employed in these sub-sectors is very difficult; establishing trends is even more uncertain. For modelling purposes we have assumed that there are around 7,800 nurses employed in these other sectors[15] and that the numbers will grow at the average (1 per cent) of the other sectors.

8.3 A forward look — the 'baseline' scenario

This section uses simulation modelling to examine the implications for intakes to pre-registration education of holding constant the labour market dynamics described in Chapter Two, together with the nurse demand assumptions outlined above, and projecting them forward for the next twenty years. This analysis provides baseline data against which we can compare (see section 8.4) alternative futures resulting from different policy interventions and labour market behaviours.

One of the most significant developments revealed by this initial projection is the ageing of the nursing workforce over the next twenty years (Figure 8.1).

By the turn of the century, the model estimates that almost half (49 per cent) the nursing workforce in Great Britain will be aged over 40 (compared with 45 per cent now). This proportion rises to nearly 53 per cent by the year 2010 when a fifth of all nurses will be aged over 50.

In this projection, the level of retirements will grow from around 5,500 a year in the late 1990s to over 10,000 a year by the middle of the next decade.

As a consequence, in order to maintain numbers, the number of new registrants entering employment would have to rise from an average of 21,000 a year between 1995 and 2005 to an average of 24,600 between 2005 and 2015 (Figure 8.2).

In order to meet this demand the required level of intakes to pre-registration nurse education would have to rise from around 24,000 in 1997/98 to 31,000 by 2011/12 (Figure 8.3). This projection assumes that there is no change in the level of discontinuations from education.

Figure 8.1 Registered nurses (wte) actual (1995) and forecast (2010) age distributions (Great Britain)

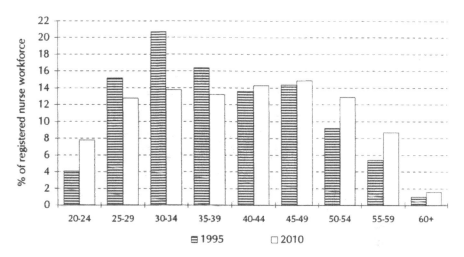

Figure 8.2 Number (wte) of newly qualified entrants required to meet demand at current growth rates, 1997/98 to 2014/15 (Great Britain)

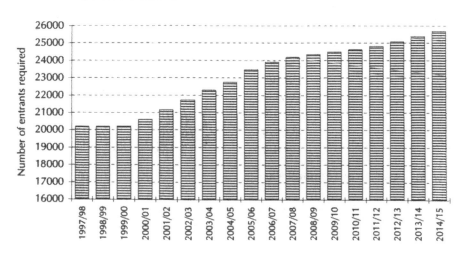

Figure 8.3 Projected intakes to pre-registration nurse education with current growth (0.7 per cent), 1997/98 to 2011/12 (Great Britain)

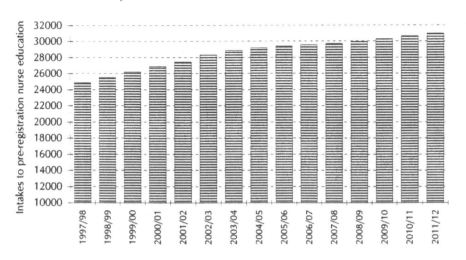

These projected entries can be compared with actual intakes to pre-registration education and training in recent years. These are shown in Table 8.1.

Table 8.1 Entries to pre-registration nursing courses in Great Britain, 1987/88 to 1995/96

Year	Entries
1987/88	22,204
1988/89	22,713
1989/90	21,335
1990/91	20,319
1991/92	20,745
1992/93	20,107
1993/94	16,242
1994/95	13,568

Source: Seccombe and Smith, 1996

The projected intakes are roughly double the size of actual intakes in the most recent years, although they are very similar to actual intakes in the late 1980s.

In practice the recent reduction in pre-registration entries is now being reversed. Forecast education commissions (including degrees, conversion and post-registration qualifications) for 1996/97 are around 14 per cent higher (for England) than in 1995/96.

The NHS Executive has indicated that '*A further substantial increase in training will be needed if future demand for qualified nurses grows*' (EL(96)45 June 1996). The Executive Letter issued in June 1996, suggests that early results from its national workforce modelling project indicate that an additional 4,000 training places for 'basic nurse training' will need to be commissioned nationally, to match the forecast demand from 2001. It suggests that increasing commissions by about 12.5 per cent in 1997/98 and again in 1998/99, should provide '*sufficient newly qualified nurses to meet demand across the healthcare sector into the next century*'.

The number of returners will also need to rise if the balance of entries to the nursing workforce is to remain at its comparatively stable historic ratio of 75 per cent newly qualified recruits to 25 per cent returners and others (*eg* overseas entrants). These projections show an increase from around 7,775 per annum over the next ten years to an average of 9,100 between 2005 and 2015.

8.4 Alternative futures

The objective of this section is to examine the effect on intakes to pre-registration nurse education of changing several of our assumptions about the future dynamics of the nursing labour market. In particular we will examine the following scenarios:

Firstly, changing retirement ages. There is unpublished evidence (from the NHS Pensions Agency) that the average age on retirement of nurses may be rising. Our first alternative scenario (the 'ageing workforce' scenario) examines the implications of a rise in the average age on retirement to 60.

Secondly, increasing the rate at which nurses return to nursing. Policy interventions designed to improve retention and return rates have always been amongst the first solutions identified by nurse workforce planners to perceived recruitment problems. Our second alternative (the 'returner' scenario) examines the effects on intakes to pre-registration education of strategies which would increase the proportion of recruits drawn from the pool from 25 per cent to 35 per cent.

Thirdly, we look at alternative demand scenarios. In the first case we consider the effect of maintaining the nursing workforce at its current level — the 'zero growth' scenario. In the second of these alternative demand scenarios, we project growth in NHS nursing employment at its long-term historic rate (2.7 per cent a year). This is our 'high growth' scenario.

Finally, we look at the effects of changing the drop-out rates from pre-registration nurse education.

8.4.1 The 'ageing workforce' scenario

If we relax our assumptions on early retirement, and assume that the average age for retirement was to increase to 60[16], the requirement for increases in intakes to training are reduced, but only marginally. That is, by the end of the period, intakes will be reduced by around 2 per cent on our baseline projection. Figure 8.4 shows the required intakes to pre-registration training required under this scenario and compares them with the 'baseline' scenario.

Figure 8.4 Projected intakes to pre-registration nurse education under baseline and 'ageing' scenarios, 1997/98 to 2011/12 (Great Britain)

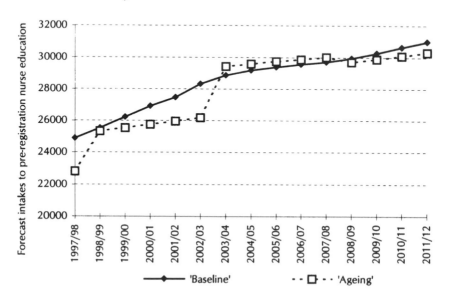

At the same time, the ageing of the nursing workforce will be more marked, with the proportion aged over 40 rising to 51 per cent by 2000/01 and to 54 per cent by 2010/11.

The ageing of the nursing workforce may, in itself, affect participation rates. Evidence from the IES/RCN membership surveys suggests that older nurses are more likely to work part-time, to work fewer part-time hours and are less likely to work beyond their contracted hours (Seccombe and Smith, 1996). A reduction in participation as a consequence of ageing could offset much of the gain from a rising age on retirement.

8.4.2 The 'returner' scenario

In this projection we have assumed that employers successfully implement a range of initiatives to encourage those nurses currently outwith nursing to return to practice. Those initiatives identified in the OPCS study (Lader, 1995) as making the greatest difference in encouraging or enabling respondents to return to work included:

- greater availability of part-time work, more flexible working hours or job sharing;

- refresher courses including updating in recent developments;

- less bureaucracy and more contact with clients/patients;

- opportunities to acquaint or reacquaint yourself with nursing before making a long term commitment;

- better resources to do the job; and

- more opportunities for developing skills.

In this projection we have increased the contribution which returners make to recruitment into the nursing workforce from 25 per cent to 35 per cent (with demand kept at its historic rate 0.7 per cent and retirement at age 60). This has the effect of further ageing the nursing workforce, projecting 57 per cent aged 40 and over by 2010 and 28 per cent aged 50 and over.

The result is that intakes to pre-registration education are reduced by about 18 per cent over the first five years of the projection period (for modelling purposes it has been assumed that the contribution rises to 35 per cent with immediate effect).

Figure 8.5 compares projected intakes to pre-registration education under the 'baseline' and 'returner' scenarios.

Figure 8.5 Projected intakes to pre-registration nurse education under baseline and returner scenarios, 1997/98 to 2011/12 (Great Britain)

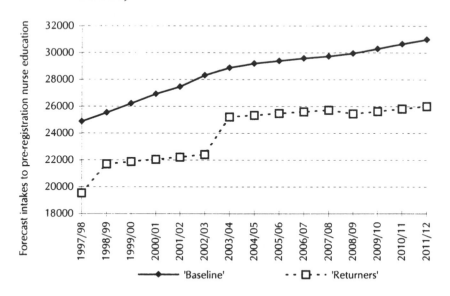

8.4.3 'Zero growth' scenario

The model can also be run under zero growth assumptions, that is, we hold the size of the nursing workforce constant at its 1995 level. This projection tells us how large intakes to education (and returner flows) would have to be to cover losses from retirement and other forms of wastage.

Figure 8.6 shows that even under these conditions, intakes to education would have to rise from 21,300 to nearly 23,700 by 2011/12 just to maintain 1995 levels. These intakes peak around 2004/05 as the effects of increasing retirements become apparent.

8.4.4 'High growth' scenario

Achieving a growth rate in nurse staffing closer to the long term historic NHS rate of 2.7 per cent would require a huge increase in the number of newly qualified nurses entering the workforce (equivalent in fact to around 7 per cent of the workforce each year). In order to achieve this, the model projects an intake to pre-registration nurse education of almost 34,800 in 1997/98, rising to more than 40,000 by 2001/02 (see Figure 8.7).

Figure 8.6 **Forecast intakes to pre-registration nurse education under baseline and 'zero growth' scenarios, 1997/98 to 2011/12 (Great Britain)**

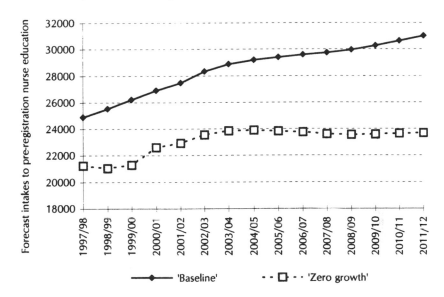

Figure 8.7 **Forecast intakes to pre-registration nurse education under baseline and '2.7 per cent growth' scenarios**

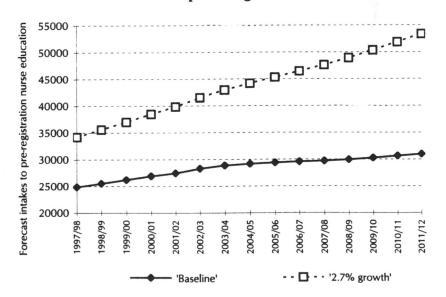

8.4.5 'Student wastage' scenario

Finally in this section we need to consider the effects of changing our assumptions about wastage from pre-registration nurse education. Hitherto our projections have applied a rate of drop-out from nurse education of 15 per cent since this was the figure recommended by the NHS Executive in its guidance to Trusts[17]. In practice, more recent evidence suggests that drop-out rates from diploma courses may be higher. Figures for England show that 23 per cent of entrants dropped out in 1994-95[18].

Projecting intakes to education assuming a 20 per cent drop-out rate increases initial entries in our base case model by around 6 per cent a year. That is, the required output to meet the baseline growth assumptions would be achieved with an intake of, for example, 28,600 in 2000/2001 compared with 26,900. A 23 per cent drop-out would require a 10 per cent increase in intakes each year, that is, 29,700 in 2000/2001 (Figure 8.8).

Figure 8.8 Projected intakes to pre-registration nurse education under baseline and 'alternative drop-out rate' scenarios, 1997/98 to 2011/12 (Great Britain)

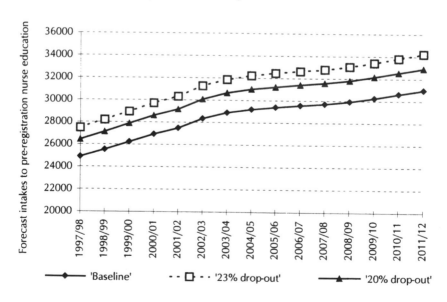

We could speculate that through the contracting process, the Education and Training Consortia (ETC) may apply greater pressure on the education providers to improve on this performance. If the average rate of drop-out could be reduced to 10 per cent, the required output (for the baseline projection) would be achieved with an intake of 25,400 in 2000/2001.

8.5 Summary and conclusions

In summary, these projections suggest that current intakes to pre-registration nurse education are barely sufficient to cope with very low growth in demand and make no allowance for any pre-existing shortfall. Intakes will also be sensitive to any changes in retirement patterns, as the overall nursing workforce ages.

Levels of intake to education are particularly sensitive to projected demand. Even with modest assumptions about growth, substantial increases in student intakes would be required. These will impose considerable pressures on costs.

In the short term, little can be done (other than reducing drop-outs from education) to alter significantly the projected outputs from pre-registration nurse education. Intakes to education have already been determined for the period to the end of the decade. Necessary increases in the nursing workforce must therefore be achieved through a combination of improved retention and return rates, and higher participation of those working part-time.

Lower drop-out rates, combined with an increase in the average age on retirement and higher labour market participation, through increasing the proportion of nurses returning to practise could offer a solution to the potential shortfall of nurses which is projected under the scenarios considered above.

However, it is also stressed that the ageing of the nursing workforce will bring other pressures, which would be particularly prominent if the retirement age was increased. Currently, older nurses are more likely to work part time, and to work shorter hours than younger nurses.

Perhaps the most significant conclusion from this exercise is the need to ensure that longer term labour market trends are taken into account when ETCs are commissioning education places, and that they are not simply projecting forward short term conditions. Otherwise, there is the clear danger that short term savings on education will be overwhelmed by the larger, long term costs of nurse shortages.

9 Conclusions

The nursing workforce is at the core of modern health services, and is a major source of employment in the UK labour market. Despite its size and importance, the characteristics and motivation of the individuals that comprise that workforce have often been misunderstood or misinterpreted. This has been largely as a result of the continued, misleading picture of the typical nurse as being young, female, single and unquestionably committed to a vocation as doctors' handmaidens. This book has attempted to correct this misleading picture and to provide a comprehensive overview of the dynamics of the UK nursing labour market and the profile of the individuals participating in that labour market.

The complexity of the UK nursing labour market, with the growth of non-NHS employment, the high levels of job mobility, the changing career prospects and paths, and the ageing of the workforce have all been given detailed consideration. The implications for policy makers of the increasing complexity of the nursing labour market have also been highlighted.

It is apparent that the need to maintain a comprehensive overview of the dynamics of the nurse labour market is greater than ever, at a time when the NHS reforms of the last decade have in some ways made establishing such an overview more difficult than before. NHS data coverage in this vital area is eroding, to the extent that the Review Body has voiced its concern that adequate nurse work force planning is under threat.

The history of nursing labour markets in Britain, and in other developed countries such as the US, is one of cycles of nursing shortages. Each shortage brings with it a horde of proposed solutions, some of which, independent evaluation strongly suggests, will have a beneficial impact.

The main interventions, highlighted in this book include:

- a systematic attempt to encourage 'returners' — acknowledging the reasons for leaving nursing, and what is required to encourage their return, but also noting the 'pool' of actual returners is probably much smaller than calculated by the Department of Health;

- the utilisation of skilled nursing staff in a way which maximises their contribution, by using appropriate and flexible working patterns;

- determining the 'right' skill mix for specific situations, taking into account quality and outcomes considerations;

- the matching of staffing levels to estimates of demand — at local *and* national level; and

- improving retention by the maintenance of career paths which encourage continual updating of skills, facilitate 'time out' of employment for other responsibilities, and provide adequate reward to individuals.

We make no claim to originality in endorsing these interventions as key factors in improving the efficiency of the nurse labour market, the effectiveness of individual nurses and the commitment of those individuals to remain in nursing. The policy reports highlighted in Appendix 1 have been promoting some of these solutions since — or before — the NHS was established in 1948. What has been missing has been a sustained attempt to implement these policy solutions within a consistent strategic framework, linked to effective integrated workforce planning. Lessons have not been learned, mistakes have been repeated, and the cycle has continued.

In specific terms, some of the main factors which deserve detailed consideration include:

- evaluation and support for widespread introduction of 'nurse-friendly' and 'family friendly' flexible working practices, with an emphasis on self scheduling;

- support for clinical career structures or 'ladders', and linked pay systems, which sustain long-term career development in clinical settings, encourage continuing education and professional development (linked to PREP) and facilitate performance review (with an emphasis on peer and professional review);

- proper recognition, within NHS career structures, of relevant non-NHS and non-nursing expertise, and mechanisms for sustaining planned career breaks;

- greater effort being given to investigating and evaluating the links between staff mix, organisational characteristics, and health outcomes; and

- improvements in data provision, locally and nationally, to enable integrated workforce planning to function effectively, and a commitment from the NHS to make such data available for planning.

The mechanisms in place in recent years have been characterised by local level planning, sometimes conducted in policy isolation from other local employers and labour markets, counterpointed by occasional knee-jerk policy interventions at national level when policy drift could no longer be sustained. This has happened most recently in the sudden government uplift in funding for education places, some time after it had become clear that the aggregate of local level decisions was leading to significant under-supply of new nursing staff. It is likely that we will continue to make the mistakes of the past until there are proper mechanisms for maintaining a national overview of the nursing labour market, linked to a participative forum formed of interested parties from the health departments, education consortia, employers and the profession.

Justification for the establishment of such a forum stems from the costly, and potentially damaging, results of not taking a more strategic overview of this important labour market. That such a forum exists to assist with the planning of the medical workforce, but has not been established for the nurse labour market is indefensible — particularly given the increasing inter-dependence of medical, nursing and other health care staff. Decisions on the employment and deployment of these staff will increasingly have to be integrated, and based on assessment of patterns of demand, and desired health outcomes. The nurse labour force is a national asset, and it requires and deserves sustained policy attention at a national level.

Notes

[1] Hereafter, the term registered nurse refers to any registered practitioner on the UKCC Register.

[2] The United Kingdom comprises England, Scotland, Wales and Northern Ireland. There are data differences between the four countries which mean that some aggregation to UK level is not feasible. In some cases, data aggregated to the level of Great Britain (GB) is used (England, Scotland and Wales).

[3] 'Pay claim will cost NHS £30m', *British Medical Journal*, vol. 314, 12 April 1997, p.1067.

[4] It is not possible to calculate a participation rate for men in all forms of nursing employment from the data published in the report.

[5] In order to provide an age distribution of practitioners living in England in 1991 we have made two assumptions: (i) the age distribution is the same as that for all practitioners, (ii) the proportion of practitioners living in England but with no postcode reported is the same as that for the Register as a whole.

[6] *Nursing Times*, 2nd October 1996, p.16.

[7] Hansard, 11/11/96, column 40.

[8] The usual convention in calculating leaver rates is to use an average staff in post figure for the year as the denominator, rather than the year end staff in post figure as reported by the OME.

[9] These are defined as nurse managers and first level registered nurses in paediatrics, maternity, community, psychiatric and learning disabilities nursing.

[10] *Nursing Standard*, 2/10/1996, p. 16.

[11] MMSAC became the Medical Workforce Standing Advisory Committee (MWSAC) in February 1995.

[12] Yorkshire Health, *Balance Sheet Guidelines 1994/95*, p. 1.

[13] The new arrangements were published in EL(95)27.

[14] Note that, because of data limitations, these forecasts are for GB rather than UK.

[15] This brings total employment in the base year for the projection to approximately 371,700 wte, which is broadly in line with the LFS total (Spring, March to May 1996).

[16] Normal retirement for most members of the NHS Pension Scheme is at age 60. Members of the special classes (including those nurses, midwives and health visitors who joined the scheme before 6 March 1995) have special retirement rights enabling them to retire with benefits from the age of 55. Unpublished data from the NHS Pensions Agency suggests that the average age on retirement for nurses has increased from 58-59.

---

[17]   *Nursing Standard*, 2/10/96, p. 16.

[18]   *Nursing Times*, 11/12/96, p. 21.

References

Advisory, Conciliation and Arbitration Service (ACAS) (1987) *Labour Flexibility in Britain*, Occasional Paper No 41, ACAS, London

Aiken L, Smith H, Lake E (1994) 'Lower Medicare mortality amongst a set of hospitals known for good nursing care', *Medical Care*, Vol. 32, pp. 771-787

Atkin K, Lunt N, Parker G, Hirst M (1993) *Nurses Count: A National Census of Practice Nurses*, Policy Research Unit, University of York

Atkinson J, Meager N (1986) *New Forms of Work Organisation*, Institute of Manpower Studies, Report 121

Audit Commission (1997) *Finders Keepers: the Management of Staff Turnover in NHS Trusts*, HMSO

Auld M (1967) 'An Investigation into the Recruitment of Part Time Nursing Staff in Hospitals', *International Journal of Nursing Studies*, Vol. 14, pp. 119-169

Bach S, Winchester D (1994) 'Opting out of pay evaluation? The prospects for local pay in UK public services', *British Journal of Industrial Relations*, Vol. 32(2), pp. 263-282

Bacon N, Kun P (1986) 'Long Shifts: A Trial Evaluated', *Australian Nurses Journal* Vol. 16, No 4, pp. 44-46

Ball J, Diskin S, Dixon M, Wyat E S (1995) *Creative Career Paths in the NHS, Report No. 4: Senior Nurses*, NHS Women's Unit, Leeds, NHS Executive

Barton J (1994) 'Shift systems in England and Wales', *Nursing Times*, Vol. 90, No. 21, p. 12

Barton J, Spelten E, Smith L, Totterdell P, Folkard S (1993) 'A Classification of Nursing and Midwifery Shift Systems', *International Journal of Nursing Studies*, Vol. 30, No 1, pp. 65-80

Beardshaw V, Robinson R (1990) *New for Old: Prospects for Nursing in the 1990s*, London: Kings Fund Institute

Becker E, Sloan F, Steinwald B (1982) 'Union Activity in Hospitals: Past, Present, Future', *Health Care Financing Review*, Vol. (4), pp. 1-13

Beishon S, Virdee S, Hagell A (1995) *Nursing in a multi-ethnic NHS*, London: Policy Studies Institute

Blegen M (1993) 'Nurses Job Satisfaction: A Meta Analysis of Related Variables', *Nursing Research*, Vol. 42 (1), pp. 36-41

Bone M R (1995) *Health expectancy and its uses*, London: HMSO

Booton C, Lane J (1985) 'Hospital Market Structure and the Return to Nursing Education', *Journal of Human Resources*, Vol. 20 (2), pp. 184-196

Brider P (1991) 'Solid Gains Behind, Leaner Times Ahead', *American Journal of Nursing*, Vol. 92, February

Briggs A (1972) *Report of the Committee on Nursing*, HMSO

Buchan J (1988) 'The Hidden Costs of the Pay Rise', *Nursing Times*, Vol. 84 (18), p. 18

Buchan J (1989) 'Regional Anomalies', *Nursing Standard*, Vol. 3 (45), p. 20

Buchan J, Seccombe I (1991) *Nurse Turnover Costs*, IES Report 212

Buchan J (1992) *Flexibility or Fragmentation: trends and prospects in nurses' pay*, London: Kings Fund Institute

Buchan J (1994a) 'Lessons from America?: US magnet hospitals and their implications for UK nursing', *Journal of Advanced Nursing*, Vol. 19, pp. 373-384

Buchan J (1994b) *Further Flexing?: NHS Trusts and Changing Working Patterns in NHS Nursing*, RCN/Queen Margaret College

Buchan J (1994c) 'The Introduction of Annualised Hours', *Nursing Standard*, Vol. 8, 18th May, p. 29

Buchan J (1996) 'The Truth Behind the Nursing Headcount', *Employing Nurses*, Vol. 10, pp. 6-7

Buchan J (1997) 'Clinical Ladders: The Ups and Downs' *International Nursing Review*, Vol. 44, No. 2., pp. 41-46.

Buchan J, Ball J (1991) *Caring Costs: Nursing Costs and Benefits*, IMS Report No. 208

Buchan J, Thomas S (1994) *Bank Nurses in Scotland: Policy and Practice*, Scottish Office

Buchan J, Seccombe I, Ball J (1992) *International Mobility of Nurses: a UK Perspective*, IMS Report 230

Buchan J, Seccombe I, Ball J (1996) *Caring Costs Revisited*, IES Report 321

Buchan J, Seccombe I, Thomas S (1997) 'Overseas Mobility of UK Nurses', *International Journal of Nursing Studies, Vol. 34, No. 1, pp. 54-62*

Buchan J, Thompson M (1997) *Recruiting, Retaining and Motivating Nurses: The use of Clinical Ladders*, Institute for Employment Studies, Report 339

Buchan J, Waite R, Thomas J (1989) *Grade Expectations: Clinical Grading and Nurse Mobility*, Institute of Manpower Studies, Report 176

Buerhaus P (1991) 'Dynamic Shortages of Registered Nurses', *Nursing Economics*, Vol. 9 (5), pp. 317-328

Buerhaus P (1993) 'Effects of RN Wages and Non Wage Income on the Performance of Hospital RN Labor Market', *Nursing Economics*, Vol. 11 (3), pp. 129-135

Carr-Hill R, Dixon P, Gibbs I, McCaughan D, Griffiths M, Wright K (1992) *Skill Mix and Effectiveness of Nursing Care*, Centre for Health Economics, University of York

Choi T, Jameson H, Brekke M (1986) 'Effects on Nurse Retention: An Experiment with Scheduling' *Medical Care*, Vol. 24, pp. 1029-1043

Clegg (1980) *Standing Commission on Pay Comparability: Nurses and Midwives*, HMSO

Cleland V (1990) *The Economics of Nursing*, Connecticut: Appleton and Lange

Conroy M, Stidston M (1988) *2001 — The Black Hole: an Examination of Labour Market Trends in Relation to the NHS*, NHS, Regional Manpower Planners Group

Cowart M, Speake D (1992) 'Supplemental Nursing Staff' in Cowart M, Serow W (eds) *'Nurses in the Workplace'*, Sage Publications, California, USA

Davies C (1990) *Collapse of the Conventional Career*, London: ENB

Department of Health (1989) *Working for Patients: Education and Training Working Paper 10*, HMSO

Department of Health (1996a) *Statistical bulletin, NHS Hospital activity statistics: England 1985 to 1995/96*, Government Statistical Office

Department of Health (1996b) *Statistical bulletin: NHS hospital and community health service non-medical staff in England, 1985-1995*, Government Statistical Office

Department of Health (1996c) *Memorandum for the Health Committee: Nursing and Midwifery Training and Staffing*

Department of Health (1997) *Statistical bulletin: NHS hospital and community health services non-medical staff in England:* 30 September 1996, Government Statistical Office

Dison C, Carter N, Bromley P (1981) 'Making the Change to Flexitime', *American Journal of Nursing*, Vol. 18, December 1981, pp. 2162-2164

Dixon M, Wyatt S, Disken S (1994) *Creating Career Paths in the NHS Report No. 2: Managers who have left the NHS, NHS Women's Unit*, NHS Executive

Dunnell K (1995) 'Population review 2: are we healthier?', *Population Trends*, Vol. 82, pp. 12-18

Dyson R (1991) 'Changing Labour Utilisation in NHS Trusts' *Trust Network*, NHS Management Executive, September

Edmonstone J (1995) 'A step into the unknown?. The new education and training contracting arrangements', *Health Manpower Management*, Vol. 21, No. 6.

EL (95) 68, *Priorities and Planning Guidance for the NHS: 1996/97*, NHS Executive, June 1995

EL (95) 96, *Non-medical education and training — planning guidance for 1996/97: education commissioning*, NHS Executive, August 1995

EL (96) 45, *Priorities and Planning Guidance for the NHS: 1997/98*, NHS Executive, June 1996

Elias P (1985) *The Distribution of Persons with Nursing Qualifications in England and Wales*, Institute for Employment Research, University of Warwick

Elliot R, Duffus K (1996) 'What Has Been Happening to Pay in the Public Service of the British Economy?', *British Journal of Industrial Relations*, Vol. 34 (1), pp. 51-85

English National Board (1997) *Annual Report 1996-97*, English National Board, London

Fields N, Loveridge C (1988) 'Critical Thinking and Fatigue: How do Nurses on 8 and 12 hours shifts compare?' *Nursing Economics*, Vol. 6, No 4, pp. 189-191

Friss L (1987) 'External Equity and the Free Market Myth', *Review of Public Personnel Administration*, Vol. 7(3), pp. 74-91

Gray A (1989) 'Nurses' Pay and the History of the NHS', *Bulletin of the History of Nursing*, Vol. 8 (2), pp. 15-27

Gray A, Phillips V (1996) Labour Turnover in the British National Health Service: A Local Labour Market Analysis, *Health Policy*, Vol. 36, pp. 273-289

Gray A, Normand C, Currie E (1988) *Staff Turnover in the NHS: A Preliminary Economic Analysis*, Discussion Paper 46. Centre for Health Economics: University of York, York

Gray A, Phillips V, Normand C (1996) 'The Costs of Nursing Turnover: Evidence from the British National Health Service', *Health Policy*, Vol. 38, pp. 117-128

Griffiths R (1983) *NHS Management Enquiry*, DHSS

Halsbury (1974) *Committee of Inquiry into the Pay and Related Conditions of Service of Nurses and Midwives*, HMSO

Handy C (1995) *The Age of Unreason*, Arrow Books

Hanson A *et al* (1997) 'Can the NHS cope in future?', *British Medical Journal*, Vol. 314, 11 January, p. 110

Harrison A, Dixon J, New B, Judge K (1997) 'Can the NHS cope in future?, *British Medical Journal*, Vol. 314, 11 January, pp. 139-42

Hirsch B, Schumacher, E (1995) 'Monopsony Power and Relative Wages in the Labor Market for Nurses', *Journal of Health Economics*, Vol. 14, pp. 443- 476

Hockey L (1976) *Women in Nursing*, Hodder and Stoughton

Hoskins M (1982) *The Effect of Pay Changes on Cohort Survival: A Study of the Supply of Midwifery Staff to the NHS*, Discussion Paper 26, Department of Economics: University of Leicester, Leicester

Hutt R, Connor II, Hirsh W (1985) *The Manpower Implications of Possible Changes in Basic Nursing Training: a Report for the RCN's Commission on Nursing Education*, IMS

Incomes Data Services (1993) *Annualised Hours*, Study No 544, IDS, London

Incomes Data Services (1994) *Derby City General Hospital NHS Trust*, Report No 667, June, p. 22, IDS, London

Irvine D, Evans M (1992) *Job satisfaction and turnover analysis among nurses: a review and meta-analysis*, Quality of Nursing Worklife Research Unit, University of Toronto/McMaster University

Irvine D, Evans M (1995) 'Job Satisfaction and Turnover Among Nurses: Integrating Research Findings Across Studies', *Nursing Research*, Vol. 44 (4), pp. 246-253

Jackson A, Eve A, (eds) (1996) *Directory of Hospice and Palliative Care Services in the UK and Republic of Ireland*, London: Hospice Information Service

Jones J, Brown R (1986) 'A Survey of the 12-hour Shift in 26 North Carolina Hospitals', *Nursing Management*, Vol. 17, May, 27-38

Lader D (1995) *Qualified Nurses, Midwives and Health Visitors*, London: OPCS

Laing and Buisson (1995) *Laing's Review of Private Healthcare 1995*, Laing and Buisson

Lancet (1932) *The Lancet Commission on Nursing*: London

Link C, Landon J (1975) 'Monopsony and Union Power in the Market for Nurses', *Southern Economic Journal*, 41 (4), pp. 649-59

Local Government Management Board (1997) *Independent Sector Workforce Survey: Residential homes and nursing homes in Great Britain,* 1996, LGMB

Long A, Mercer G (1981) *Manpower Planning in the National Health Service,* Gower

McCarthy W E J (1976) *Making Whitley Work: a Review of the Operation of the National Health Service and Whitley Council Systems,* HMSO

Medical Workforce Standing Advisory Committee (1995) *Planning the Medical Workforce: second report,* Department of Health

Miller M (1984) 'Implementing Self Scheduling' *Journal of Nursing Administration,* Vol. 14, No 3, pp. 33-36

Miller R, Becker B, Krinsky E (1979) *The Impact of Collective Bargaining on Hospitals,* Praeger: New York

Ministry of Health (1939) *Inter-departmental Committee on Nursing Services: Interim Report*

Ministry of Health (1947) *Report of the Working Party on the Recruitment and Training of Nurses,* HMSO

Ministry of Health (1957) *Report of the Committee to Consider the Future Numbers of Medical Practitioners and the Appropriate Intake of Medical Students,* (The Willink Report), HMSO

Ministry of Health and Department of Health for Scotland (1944) *Report of the Inter-Departmental Committee on Medical Schools,* (The Goodenough Report), HMSO

Moore K (1996) 'Non-medical workforce planning within a consortium model', Paper presented to Conference on *Achieving organisational change through workforce planning,* Royal College of Surgeons, London, 28 March 1996

Moores B, Singh B, Tun A (1983) 'An Analysis of the Factors which Impinge on a Nurses' Decision to Enter, Stay in, Leave or Re-enter the Nursing Profession', *Journal of Advanced Nursing,* p. 8, pp. 227-235

Mower M, Rodgers D (1993) 'Time Machine', *Health Service Journal,* Vol. 103, 17th June, p. 37

National Audit Office (1985) *National Health Service: Control of Nursing Manpower,* HMSO

NHS Personnel (1996) *Competency Based Pay in the NHS: Resource Pack,* NHS Personnel: Sheffield

NHSE (1996) Draft Workforce Balance Sheet for 1996/97 Commissions

North West Thames Regional Health Authority, Pay and Manpower Unit (1992) *Where's the Fat in Whitley?,* North West Thames RHA.

O'Byrne J (1989) 'Working Flexitime', *Nursing Standard,* Vol. 3, No 38

O'Connor T, (1992) 'Twelve Hour Shifts Begin in Dunedin' *New Zealand Nurses Journal*, Vol. 85, No 10. pp. 20-21

Office of Health Economics (1995) *Compendium of Health Statistics*, (9th Edition), London: OHE

Palmer J (1991) 'Eight and Twelve Hour Shifts: Comparing Nurses' Behaviour Patterns', *Nursing Management*, Vol. 22, No 9, pp. 42-44

Phillips, V (1995) 'Nurses' Labor Supply: Participation, Hours of Work, and Discontinuities in the Supply Function', *Journal of Health Economics*, Vol. 14, pp. 567-582

Price Waterhouse (1987) *Report on the Cost, Benefits and Manpower Implications of Project 2000*, UKCC

Pudney S, Shield M (1997) 'Gender, race, pay and promotion in the British nursing profession: estimation of a generalised order profit model', *Unpublished paper*, University of Leicester

RCN (1985) *Commission on Nursing Education: The Education of Nurses: a New Dispensation*, (The Judge Commission)

Reid N, Robinson G, Todd C (1993) 'The Quantity of Nursing Care on Wards working 8 and 12-hour shifts', *International Journal of Nursing Studies*, Vol. 3, No 5, pp. 403-413

Reid N, Robinson G, Todd C (1994) 'The 12 hour Shift: the views of nurse educators and students', *Journal of Advanced Nursing*, Vol. 19, No 5, pp. 938-946

Reid N, Todd C, Robinson G (1991) 'Educational Activities on Wards under 12 Hour Shifts', *International Journal of Nursing Studies*, Vol. 28, No 1, pp. 47-54

Review Body for Nursing Staff, Midwives, Health Visitors and Professions Allied to Medicine, *Report on Nursing Staff, Midwives and Health Visitors*, (various years), Stationery Office

Richardson G, Maynard A (1995) *Fewer Doctors? More Nurses?: A Review of the Knowledge Base of Doctor-Nurse Substitution*, Centre for Health Economics, Discussion Paper 15, University of York

Royal Commission (1968) *Royal Commission on Medical Education 1965-68*, The Todd Report, HMSO

Sadler J, Whitworth T (1975) *Reserves of Nurses*, London: OPCS

Scottish Office (1997) *Student Nurse Numbers: Report of the Steering Group on Student Nurse Intake Assessment*, Scottish Office Department of Health, Edinburgh

Seccombe I, Buchan J (1991) *Nurse Turnover Costs*, IMS Report 212

Seccombe I, Buchan J (1993) *Absent Nurses: The Costs and Consequences*, IES Report 250

Seccombe I, Buchan J (1994) 'The Changing Role of The NHS Personnel Function' Robinson R; LeGrand J. *Evaluating the NHS Reforms*, London: Kings Fund

Seccombe I, Patch A (1995) *Recruiting, Rewarding and Retaining Qualified Nurses in 1995*, IES Report 295

Seccombe I, Smith G (1996) *In the Balance: Registered Nurse Supply and Demand, 1996* Institute for Employment Studies, IES Report No. 315

Seccombe I, Smith G (1997a) *Taking Part: Registered Nurses and the Labour Market in 1997*, IES Report 338

Seccombe I, Smith G (1997b) *Taking part: Registered Nurses and the Labour Market in 1997*, a Summary for the Pay Review Body, IES Report 338

Seccombe I, Smith G, Buchan J, Ball J (1997) *Enrolled nurses: a study for the UKCC*, IES Report 344

Seccombe I, Jackson C, Patch A (1995) *Nursing: the Next Generation*, IES Report 274

Seccombe I, Patch A, Stock J (1994) *Workload, Pay and Morale of Qualified Nurses in 1994*, IES Report 272

Seccombe I, Ball J, Patch A (1993) *The Price of Commitment: Nurses Pay, Careers and Prospects*, Institute of Manpower Studies, Report 251

Secretaries of State (1989) *Working for Patients*, HMSO

Thompson M, Buchan J (1993) *Performance Related Pay and UK Nursing*, IMS Report No. 235

Todd C, Reid N, Robinson G (1989) 'The Quality of Nursing Care on Wards Working Eight and Twelve Hour Shifts', *International Journal of Nursing Studies*, Vol. 26, No 4, pp. 359-368

UKCC (1996) *Statistical Analysis of the Council's Professional Register, 1 April 1995 to 31 March 1996*, UKCC

Waite R, Hutt R (1987) *Attitudes, Jobs and Mobility of Qualified Nurses*, IMS Report 130

Waite R, Buchan J, Thomas J (1989) *Nurses in and out of Work*, IMS Report No. 170

Waite R, Buchan J, Thomas J (1990) *Career Patterns of Scotland's Qualified Nurses*, Scottish Office

Wilson R, Stilwell J (1992) *The National Health Service and the Labour Market*, England: Avebury Press

Wunderlich G, Sloan S, Davis C (eds) (1996) *Nursing Staff in Hospitals and Nursing Homes: is it Adequate?*, Washington DC: Institute of Medicine, National Academy Press

Yett D (1970) *An Economic Analysis of the Nursing Shortage*, Lexington, Massachusetts: D C Heath

Appendix 1: Previous Reports of UK Nursing Shortages

The Lancet Commission on Nursing published in 1932, to *'inquire into the reasons for the shortage of candidates, trained and untrained, for nursing the sick '.*

The Commission examined vacancy rates, turnover rates, application rates and level of advertisements in nursing journals. They also took evidence from professional organisations and hospital associations. Their recommendations (which reflect a pre-NHS health service) included proposals on salary scales; maximum permitted hours of work (including an 11 hour maximum night shift); *'universal adoption of the College of Nursing scale of minimum salaries for posts higher than that of ward sister';* reform of nurse education; provision of in-service training; *'provision of sufficient ward maids to relieve nurses of domestic duties '.*

The Inter-Departmental Committee on Nursing Services in its Interim Report (1939) were charged with *'inquiring into the arrangements at present in operation with regard to the recruitment, training and registration and terms and conditions of service of persons engaged in nursing the sick . . . '.*

The Committee referred to the *'great urgency of the problems'* (para 2) it had been asked to address, highlighted *'the paucity of reliable statistical material relating to the nursing services'* (para 3) and conducted a survey of all hospitals and employing institutions. The Committee stressed the need for nursing to be a career *'which can compete on equal terms with the many other avenues of employment now open to women'* (para 10) and argued that *'only if the two fundamental matters of salary and pension are treated on a national basis will the present condition of the profession be improved. We have been impressed by evidence given before us which shows how local authorities and other employing bodies have been forced by circumstances to compete with each other for the services of probationers and fully qualified nurses. This is good neither for the employer nor the nurse, who is encouraged to move from one hospital to another at short intervals, with effects which react adversely on the nurses work and on her patients'* (para 13).

In relation to shortages, the Committee noted that '*there exists an acute general shortage of State Registered Nurses ... the shortage is not confined to any one locality ...* ' (para 19). There had been no falling off in the number of new recruits (para 21) but 'quality' fluctuated, depending on the availability of other career opportunities, and there was an '*astonishing loss*' of first year probationers (at least 25 per cent wastage) (para 22).

The '*real cause*' of the shortage, the Committee decided, was that '*demand had far outpaced supply*' (para 25). Contributory factors included the competition of outside employment, and high marriage rates. The Committee's recommendations included: salaries and pensions to be dealt with on a national basis; central control of recruitment to nursing; restructuring of nurse education courses; reduction in hours of work; additional 'off duty' for nurses working excess hours; increase in the number of orderlies and ward maids; 'extension of the practice of employing married nurses'; universal and interchangeable pensions, (para 169).

The report of the **Ministry of Health Working Party on the Recruitment and Training of Nurses** (1947) noted *that 'the fact that the difficulties in the health service are still acute in all fields must be ascribed to the growth of the services and the consequent demand for increased staff ... '* (para 28). Once again, demand outstripping supply was being highlighted as the major problem.

The Working Party considered that '*information showing how nurses are distributed with respect to age, educational background, qualifications etc. is an indispensable part of the equipment needed for planning the profession. No such information was available when we began our inquiries and we accordingly endeavoured to fill this gap in our knowledge*' para 29.

The Working Party commissioned a survey of a random stratified sample of nurses working in 184 hospitals - some 6,600 questionnaires were completed. The survey obtained information on age profile, current occupation, educational background, career history *etc.* They also commissioned a separate study to examine mobility turnover and wastage of nursing staff, based on information from 161 hospitals. Wastage (*ie* outflow) was found to be 11-12 per cent.

The main conclusions of the Working Party were: nurses in training should have full student status; reform of nurse education; all restrictions on employment of married nurses to be removed; part time service to be developed; use of male nurses to be extended.

The report of the **Committee on Nursing** (Briggs 1972) again restated the problem of information inadequacies: 'There are no adequate data relating to the overall balance between nursing and midwifery supply and demand at national level'. They also noted that 'it is not possible to measure shortages without first establishing needs' (para 446).

Briggs (1972) acknowledged staff shortage difficulties in the staff nurse grade, and in geriatric/long stay and psychiatric settings. Another factor which had contributed to increasing demand was the reduction in the average length of stay which increased dependency levels and workload (para 480). The report included the results of surveys of nurses and employers. Main recommendations, in relation to improving the supply/demand balance, included: recruiting 'mature entrants'; recruiting male nurses; encouraging nurse returners and improving part-time opportunities; establishing 'keep in touch' scheme for nurses on maternity leave; improving shift patterns and the allocation of staff to workload; conducting opinion surveys of nurses to identify work related difficulties (paras 433-501).

Appendix 2: Participation in Nursing and Estimated Pool Size

This Appendix details how estimates were derived for participation rates and the size of the potential pool.

A2.1 Participation

Most workforce data is presented as wte numbers which have to be converted to a headcount figure. Wherever possible headcount data has been used. Where it is unavailable we have used official data sources for England to estimate the headcount. The sources used include: the Non-medical Workforce Census (NHS nurses), the GMS bi-annual return (GP practice nurses) and the KO36 annual returns (non-NHS nurses in hospitals, clinics, residential homes and nursing homes). These data suggest that the wte is 0.8 for nurses in the NHS, 0.55 for GP practice nurses and 0.77 for nurses in the non-NHS sector. The wte figures were applied to data for the rest of the UK. Estimates of the number of registered nurses in each sector is shown in Table B.1. Note that data for Northern Ireland on the number of practice nurses and nurses in the non-NHS sector is a minimum figure. The data are not held centrally, but are held by the four health and social service boards, and the Registration and Inspection Units at each area board respectively.

Evidence from the IES/RCN survey suggests that as many as four per cent of nurses work in other sectors such as armed forces, hospice care, occupational health, *etc.*:

- 480,079 × 0.04 = 19,203.

Using this approach the sum total of nurses employed in the UK is estimated to be 499,282.

Table A2.1   Estimated numbers (wte and headcount) of registered nurses employed in the UK, by employment sector

	NHS nursing	GP practice nursing		Non-NHS nursing		Total
GB	292,300 (wte)					
England		17,898	(n)	66,300	(n)	
Scotland		1,349	(n)	8,246	(n)	
Wales		621	(wte)	2,679	(wte)	
Northern Ireland	11,480 (wte)	100	(n)	1,853	(n)	
Headcount total	**379,725**	**20,476**		**79,878**		**480,079**

Source: IES/ Annual Abstract of Statistics/ KO36 return/ GMS return/ Scottish Health Statistics/ Health and Personal Social Services Statistics for Wales/ Welsh Office data/ unpublished data from the Department of Health Northern Ireland and Health and Social Services Boards

Using the number of practitioners on the UKCC Register (living in the UK) as the denominator gives a participation rate in nursing employment of 81 per cent.

A2.2 Estimated pool size

The population of registered nurses in the UK is 618,811.

- 4.4 per cent (n = 27,228) of this population are aged over 60. Some of these will be potentially unavailable for nursing work; thus potential population, from which employers can recruit, is estimated at 591,583.

If there are an estimated 499,282 registered nurses employed in nursing then the potential pool of returners is 92,301:

- survey evidence suggests that between eight and 16 per cent of nurses in this pool are employed in non-nursing work, *ie* 7,304 to 14,768;

- survey evidence suggests that historically, few of these individuals have returned to nursing work; the future career intentions of those in non-nursing work confirms this pattern.

Thus the size of the potential pool of registered nurses, available for nursing work, is likely to lie between 77,533 and 84,997.

Appendix 3: Modelling the labour market for registered nurses

The projections of intakes to pre-registration nurse education and training contained in this book are based on three models. Each is described briefly in this appendix.

Registered Nurse Demand Model

The first model, the Registered Nurse Demand Model, projects the future stock of registered nurses in each segment of the nursing labour market (NHS, GP practice, non-NHS, agency and other) on the basis of observed long term trends in staff numbers. These are aggregated to provide an overall nursing workforce figure for each year of the projection.

Nurse Workforce Model

The second model, the Nurse Workforce Model, projects the stocks and movements of registered nurses (using whole time equivalents) from a base date (1995) in Great Britain. The model begins by calculating the numbers (wte) of nurses moving out of the nursing workforce (wastage) by removing premature retirees, normal retirements and other leavers. It then compares the resulting stocks after wastage with the target number (wte) in nursing employment at the end of the 12 month period, to derive the number of vacancies to be filled.

The model then fills the vacancies from two sources.

- pre-registration education (the newly qualified flow); and

- the pool of non-working nurses (the returners flow). Note that the pool could include entries from outside Great Britain.

Vacancies are filled in the ratio 75 per cent newly qualified to 25 per cent returners, using the observed proportions from the 1995 OPCS study (Lader, 1995) and unpublished data made available from NHS sources in Scotland.

The main output from the model is the required number of newly qualified entrants to meet a given level of demand for staff. The newly qualified entrants figure provides the input to our third model.

Pre-registration Education Model

The third model, the Pre-registration Education Model, relates the number qualifying (*ie* becoming eligible to register), to the number entering an appropriate number of years earlier depending on the route to registration. It also makes allowance for the small proportion of those who qualify from pre-registration education who are eligible to register but who chose not to do.

Printed and bound by CPI Group (UK) Ltd, Croydon, CR0 4YY

21/10/2024

01777085-0004